NUTRITIONAL PROBLEMS IN A CHANGING WORLD

Proceedings of The British Nutrition Foundation Research Conference on 'Nutritional Problems in a Changing World—Nutrition in Britain Today and Tomorrow', held at Churchill College, Cambridge, 29 March–4 April 1973

NUTRITIONAL PROBLEMS
in a
CHANGING WORLD

Edited by

DOROTHY HOLLINGSWORTH
Director-General

and

MARGARET RUSSELL
Scientific Information Officer

*The British Nutrition Foundation
London, England*

A HALSTED PRESS BOOK

JOHN WILEY & SONS
New York — Toronto

PUBLISHED IN THE U.S.A. AND CANADA BY
HALSTED PRESS
A DIVISION OF JOHN WILEY & SONS, INC., NEW YORK

Library of Congress Cataloging in Publication Data

Main entry under title:
Nutritional problems in a changing world.
    "A Halsted Press book."
    Proceedings of a conference held by the British Nutrition
Foundation at Churchill College, Cambridge, Eng., Mar.
29–Apr. 4, 1973.
    1. Nutrition—Congresses.   I. Hollingsworth, Dorothy
Frances, ed.   II. Russell, Margaret, ed.   III. British
Nutrition Foundation.
TX345.N89   613.2   73-15980
ISBN: 0–470–40717–4

WITH 65 TABLES AND 29 ILLUSTRATIONS

© APPLIED SCIENCE PUBLISHERS LTD 1973

Printed in Great Britain by Galliard (Printers) Ltd, Great Yarmouth, Norfolk, England

Preface

When we were planning the programme for the BNF Research Conference we decided to consider the nutritional condition of people in an affluent society, such as Britain, not from the point of view of specific nutrients or possible specific nutritional deficiencies, but rather to assemble as much information as possible on the nutritional needs and status of people of different ages living in Britain today. We took as our base Shakespeare's seven ages of man. We wanted to be able to answer the questions 'What is the present nutritional condition of the people and is there anything new that the British Nutrition Foundation should be doing about it?'

We decided that as an overture we must review the means available today for practising nutritional surveillance and we devoted one day's discussion to this topic. We proceeded by way of infant feeding and child development to a study of the nutritional needs of adults, including consideration of whether or not food in such a country as Britain needs to be fortified with certain nutrients; this led to an attempt to answer the questions whether the elderly have special nutritional needs and whether it is possible by dietary means to halt progression from the sixth to the seventh age—that 'second childishness . . . sans everything'.

We ended with a day's discussion on the relevance of modern nutritional thought to the present problems of the food industry, consideration of gaps in today's research in nutritional sciences and, finally, to the formulation of six recommendations prepared by individual members of the Conference for review by the Council of the British Nutrition Foundation.

In designing our programme we had to be selective and we were forced by time to omit several topics of great current concern. Some of these topics were the subject of four plenary lectures which are collected as Chapters 1–4 of this book.

Part 1 records the experiences of four countries, Britain, Canada, Czechoslovakia and the United States of America, in attempting to assess the nutritional status of their respective populations.

Some of the problems of feeding infants are discussed in Part 2 and of child development in Part 3. Aspects of the nutritional requirements of adults, including the elderly, are considered in Part 4.

The relevance of modern nutritional thought for the food industry is

v

the subject of Part 5 and our reflections, conclusions and recommendations are recorded in Part 6.

The members of the various scientific committees of the British Nutrition Foundation provided many ideas for the programme of this Conference, and we should like to express our gratitude to them. We should, however, like particularly to record our especial thanks to three individual scientists: Dr W. T. C. Berry for his help in planning the sessions on nutritional surveillance; Dr E. M. Widdowson for initiating and planning the sessions on infant feeding and child development, and Dr J. P. Greaves, formerly Secretary of the British Nutrition Foundation, whose enthusiasm and knowledge were of great value during the early stages of preparing for the Conference.

DOROTHY HOLLINGSWORTH

MARGARET RUSSELL

Foreword

PROFESSOR SIR FRANK YOUNG, FRS

President, The British Nutrition Foundation

The holding of the first research Conference of the British Nutrition Foundation in March/April 1973 marked a notable step in the Foundation's evolution. Membership of the Conference was by invitation only, but each member Company had the right to nominate a representative as a member of the Conference, while a number of distinguished nutritionists and food scientists, some from abroad, were invited by the Officers of the Foundation also to take part. Some members agreed, by invitation, to present formal papers or lectures to the Conference and now all the contributed papers and lectures appear in published form under the able editorship of Miss D. F. Hollingsworth, OBE, Director-General of the British Nutrition Foundation, and Mrs M. Russell the Scientific Information Officer of the Foundation. A brief summary of certain conclusions and recommendations is also included.

For the organisation of this Conference the British Nutrition Foundation was fortunate in securing the services, as temporary Conference Organising Secretary, of Mrs Nancy Spufford, who had retired from a comparable full-time post with the Ciba Foundation, London, in the course of which she had played a large part in the organisation of numerous smaller, nonnutritional, international conferences of a similar sort. With the aid of Mrs Spufford, the Officers of the British Nutrition Foundation, and especially the Director-General, Dorothy Hollingsworth, were able to plan a programme which provided time for ample discussion, both formal and informal, and which seemed to receive general approval in practice.

The membership of the Conference included representatives of the Nutrition Foundation Inc. (USA) and of the Swedish Nutrition Foundation, and their presence helped to maintain the cooperation that is developing internationally between national Nutrition Foundations.

As President of the British Nutrition Foundation I took the Chair at the main sessions of the Conference, and otherwise assisted to fulfil the plans which had been delineated by Dorothy Hollingsworth, Nancy Spufford, and (more recently) with the aid of Margaret Russell. Unlike Paris I shall make no attempt to present a prize to any of the three Graces but I can unhesitatingly say that without their untiring and inspired planning the Conference would have lacked the scientific acumen and grace that in the end it proved to possess.

That was the first Conference of its kind run by the British Nutrition Foundation. Here are the results of the Conference, in cold print, now available for all to see and to judge.

Contents

PART 4

FOOD FOR ADULTS: HOW MUCH AND OF WHAT KIND? IS THERE A CASE FOR FORTIFICATION?

PART 5

IMPLICATIONS OF MODERN NUTRITIONAL THOUGHT FOR THE FOOD INDUSTRY

PART 6

CONCLUSIONS AND RECOMMENDATIONS

List of Contributors

R. J. L. ALLEN
   Group Research Director, Beecham Group Ltd, Beecham House, Great West Road, Brentford, Middlesex

W. T. C. BERRY
   4, Church Farm, Colney, Norwich NOR 70F

DENIS P. BURKITT
   Medical Research Council External Staff, 172, Tottenham Court Road, London W1P 9LH

W. J. H. BUTTERFIELD
   Vice-Chancellor, University of Nottingham, University Park, Nottingham NG7 2RD

SHEILA T. CALLENDER
   Consultant in Medicine, Nuffield Department of Clinical Medicine, The Radcliffe Infirmary, Oxford

J. A. CAMPBELL
   Acting Director, Nutrition Bureau, Department of National Health and Welfare, Queensway Towers, 200, Isabella Street, Ottawa, Ontario K1A 1B7, Canada

W. J. DARBY
   President, The Nutrition Foundation, Inc., 99, Park Avenue, New York, NY 10016, USA

SYLVIA J. DARKE
   Senior Medical Officer—Nutrition, Department of Health and Social Security, Alexander Fleming House, Elephant and Castle, London SE1 6BY

G. A. H. ELTON

Chief Scientific Adviser (Food), Ministry of Agriculture, Fisheries and Food, Great Westminster House, Horseferry Road, London SW1P 2AE

A. N. EXTON-SMITH

Physician, Geriatric Department, St Pancras Hospital, University College Hospital, 4, St Pancras Way, London NW1 0PE

SIR GEORGE GODBER

Chief Medical Officer, Department of Health and Social Security, Alexander Fleming House, Elephant and Castle, London SE1 6BY (also, Chief Medical Officer, Department of Education and Science)

H. GOLDSTEIN

National Children's Bureau, Adam House, 1, Fitzroy Square, London W1P 5AH

MAVIS GUNTHER

77, Ember Lane, Esher, Surrey KT10 8EG

D. M. HEGSTED

Professor of Nutrition, School of Public Health, Harvard University, 665, Huntingdon Avenue, Boston, Mass. 02115, USA

S. HEJDA

Research Centre of Metabolism and Nutrition of the Institute for Clinical and Experimental Medicine, Budějovická 800, Prague 4-Krč, Czechoslovakia

A. W. HUBBARD

Superintendent, Food and Nutrition Division, Department of Trade and Industry, Laboratory of the Government Chemist, Cornwall House, Stamford Street, London SE1 9NQ

A. T. JAMES

Colworth Welwyn Laboratory, Unilever Limited, Colworth House, Sharnbrook, Bedford

E. KODICEK

Director, Dunn Nutritional Laboratory, Milton Road, Cambridge, CB4 1XJ

J. MAŠEK
Research Centre of Metabolism and Nutrition of the Institute of Clinical and Experimental Medicine, Budějovická 800, Prague 4-Krč, Czechoslovakia

B. E. C. NORDIN
Director, Medical Research Council Mineral Metabolism Unit, The General Infirmary, Great George Street, Leeds LS1 3EX

D. S. PARSONS
Department of Biochemistry, South Parks Road, University of Oxford, Oxford OX1 3QU

EUAN M. ROSS
Department of Child Health, Royal Hospital for Sick Children, St Michael's Hill, Bristol BS2 8BJ

J. C. L. SHAW
Department of Paediatrics, University College Hospital Medical School, Huntley Street, London WC1E 6DH

H. M. SINCLAIR
Lady Place, Sutton Courtenay, Berkshire

D. A. T. SOUTHGATE
Dunn Nutritional Laboratory, Milton Road, Cambridge CB4 1XJ

A. SPICER
Director of Research, RHM Research Limited, The Lord Rank Research Centre, Lincoln Road, High Wycombe, Bucks

L. S. TAITZ
The Children's Hospital, Western Bank, Sheffield S10 2TH

A. S. TRUSWELL
Professor of Nutrition and Dietetics, Queen Elizabeth College, Atkins Building, London W8 7AH

ELSIE M. WIDDOWSON

Infant Nutrition Research Division, Dunn Nutritional Laboratory, Milton Road, Cambridge CB4 1XJ

F. WOOD

Development Director, CPC (United Kingdom) Ltd, Claygate House, Esher, Surrey KT10 9PN

CHAPTER 1

Nutrition and public health

G. E. GODBER

Chief Medical Officer, Department of Health and Social Security, London

The term public health now has a very different connotation from that which Sir John Simon, my first predecessor, would have given to it over a century ago. It is nearer to that which Sir George Newman, the first Chief Medical Officer of the newly constituted Ministry of Health would have used 53 years ago but still very different in its scope. Public health meant to Simon the kind of activity which needed medical guidance because there was no one else to provide it with impetus at all, but which was rather outside the ordinary role of the doctor. It meant a collection of services provided by local authorities, with guidance from the centre, in order to safeguard the health of the public from environmental hazards, chiefly due to specific infective agents. Indeed in the second half of the last century it went beyond action on the environment only to the extent of providing for segregation of people with communicable infections, for the safety of others rather than for their own treatment. It was a world in which roughly 1 in 7 of all babies died within a year of their birth and 1 in 250 of all women having babies died in the process. The corresponding ratios now are 1 in 55 and 1 in 7000. It was a world in which there were certainly serious nutritional deficiencies, some of which were shown all too clearly at the time of the large scale recruitment to the forces for the war in South Africa at the end of the last century. A new awareness was beginning to lead to serious attempts to improve the care of children through voluntary or local authority provided maternity and child welfare services and then the school health service; the first owing much to Sir Arthur Newsholme and the second being essentially designed by Sir George Newman. But the main contribution to the support of the destitute was still through the Poor Law up to the time of the Local Government Act of 1929 and even after that through the lineal descendant of the Poor Law, public assistance provided by Counties and County Boroughs until the National Assistance Act and the National Health Service Act both came into effect on 5 July 1948.

Maternity and child welfare services and school health services of course could hardly exist without uncovering the nutritional deficiencies suffered by so many children in the period between the wars, especially through the hard times of the early 1930s. By then our record as shown by

1

infant mortality was steadily improving, but when I was doing school medical and maternity and child welfare work 35 years ago, it was easy enough by simple clinical examination to identify malnutrition and particularly rickets in an appreciable proportion of infants and school-children.

It was a time which many of a later generation would find hard to en-visage, but it was the time when McGonigle could show in his book 'Poverty and Public Health' how damaging an exercise rehousing could be when it led to better physical surroundings, but to such an additional strain on the family budget that there was too little left to provide for food. That exercise is well known. Two slum areas, one cleared and the population rehoused on the edge of the town and the other remaining with its popula-tion still in unsatisfactory old housing, but having more money for food because rents were lower and having a demonstrably more favourable health record, as judged by death rates.

We are far from having all wants satisfied now. There are large families with young children in the lowest income groups about whom all of us who have been involved in the work of the Committee on Medical Aspects of Food Policy (COMA) have been deeply concerned; and there are old people who for one reason or another are unable to secure for themselves the minimum intake of the right food. Rickets may now be only demon-strable where there are special family circumstances which have led to a deficient intake of vitamin D, but that does not mean that all—particularly those in some immigrant groups—are getting the vitamin D that they need. A study in Birmingham published recently suggests they are not. There may not be sufficient evidence to confirm Professor Nordin's thesis that the osteoporosis occurring in too many of our old people is due to lack of vitamin D in their diets, but there are certainly 25 000 or more admissions a year to hospital because of fracture of the femoral neck. We have not come up with an alternative explanation or, for that matter, any evidence for ways of preventing so serious a drain on our health resources and so substantial a cause of illness, crippling and death. A recent study of deep body temperatures in old people and the temperatures of their living accommodation has reported that some of them need more warmth. If they lack the resources for heating, some at least of them may also lack the food they require. The deficiency may arise from mismanagement but it may still be there.

Malnutrition of course was not always due to mere deficiency of the resources to provide the necessary nutrients. It could also be due to misuse of what was available. Traditional dietary patterns, given sufficient funds, might take care of the needs of all but the very young. The successes of maternity and child welfare services were very largely the result of inculcating improved patterns of infant feeding of which Truby King was the pioneer in New Zealand, and upon which the paediatricians have since so much improved. There was a rigidity and certainty about the advice one gave the young mothers 35 years ago, but at least it was better than the mixture of grandmotherly guidance, or none at all, upon which they themselves had been brought up.

Now of course the body of traditional knowledge has been radically changed and the young mothers' clubs of today no longer need to unlearn even the kind of ritual my contemporaries and I were teaching their mothers between the wars. There is a great deal more readily accessible and sensibly written literature most of them can use and there are conveniently prepared ingredients for infant diets which make sound feeding easy enough provided you can afford them. But even in those foods there can be mistakes; the recent report on lead in food has shown that some canning methods may result in an undesirably high concentration of lead in some of them.

The 1939/45 war gave the health interests a real opportunity to provide for certain priorities. In place of a multiplicity of infant foods of widely varying cost, a national dried milk fortified with vitamin D was provided at reduced cost or free. Sufficient milk, liquid or dried, was ensured for the pregnant and nursing mother, the infant and the preschool child. Milk was provided for all schoolchildren and provision of school meals was made general. All these measures were to ensure that the age groups most at risk in time of national food shortage should be certain of having the foods they most needed. The years 1939 to 1945, because of the strain on health services, might have been expected to produce at the least a pause in the improvement in health of children as reflected in mortality rates. In fact, during the 1940s infant mortality fell twice as rapidly as in the preceding decade. And at ages 1–4 and 5–9 mortality declined even faster. Part of the improvement at later ages was due to improved control of communicable disease, but in the preschool age groups it is likely that improved nutrition was the main factor in reducing mortality, for of necessity the other health services were in no position then, from sheer lack of manpower, to make rapid progress. Perhaps the experience of that decade did as much by improving knowledge of sound dietary principles, and the effect of better nutrition may well have continued on to the present time, because the young mothers of the 1960s had better physique, the result of better nutrition in early childhood. The theoretical basis of what was done then was fairly flimsy. There had been the League of Nations and the British Medical Association series of recommended intakes of different nutrients, not based on accurate knowledge and therefore containing a margin of safety which in retrospect seems too large. We still lack accurate information about optimal intakes and still are too apt to operate on the basis of a wide safety margin if one is not sure of the optimum level, regardless of the fact that an excess of some nutrients like vitamin D can be positively damaging. In fact the record of fortification of infant foods with vitamin D is an object lesson. The original national dried milk was fortified with vitamin D as were some of the proprietary milks at the time. Additional vitamin D was considered essential beyond this and supplements of vitamins A and C were also included in the welfare food scheme. Altogether the supplements allowed for an average intake of 800 international units (iu) of vitamin D a day for an infant and in the light of present knowledge that was more than was needed even if no other food was fortified. Thereafter, on the general principle that more of what was good in milk must be better for other foods, vitamin D was added to a variety of infant foods by their makers and we ended with combined average intakes, if all the best foods were used, of considerably over the minimum requirements. If a vitamin D concentrate was then given, perhaps rather liberally, some infants might be taking 2000 or 3000 iu a day where only one-seventh of the amount would certainly have been sufficient. A few cases of hypercalcaemia were reported and a special Sub-Committee of the Standing Medical Advisory Committee had to look into the whole question of fortification before we came round to the conclusion that a limited supplement only of vitamin D was necessary and the need for this could be further reduced by the extent to which an infant was being fed on other artificially fortified foods. The fortification of dried milk had been regulated on a basis which prescribed only a minimum but no maximum level. This had to be altered and the resulting maximum was actually below the level of the minimum previously prescribed.

During the war the extraction rate of flour was *raised* to 80% or more (depending on supplies) and this provided rather more of certain nutrients than would have been the case otherwise. Calcium was also added and this continued to be added when the extraction rate was reduced again despite the fact that the original theoretical reasons for adding it no longer existed. Over the years other reasons have been advanced; whether they too will ultimately be found to be valid we do not know. This is an example of how difficult it is to take steps to reduce the intake of a nutrient unless this can actually be proved to be harmful and contrasts oddly with the difficulty of getting demonstrably necessary fluoride added to water.

From 1940 and continuing after food rationing ended, we continued to maintain a survey of food intakes upon which, using our admittedly uncertain criteria of requirements, an estimate could be made of the level of probability that malnutrition might occur. As a method it depends on a lot of assumptions about the efficient use of food bought, and about its distribution within the family. The sufficiency of various nutrients can only be calculated on the basis of recommended allowances and analyses of nutrient contents of the foods themselves. Inevitably there is a wide margin of error, but the information was the best obtainable and a great deal better than guesswork. It was the best we could do in the absence of reliable clinical or laboratory criteria of nutritional levels. Even with such other evidence as was then available it left the body of experts trying to monitor nutritional levels in a very insecure position and quite unable to reject, authoritatively, claims to identify borderline deficiency states. One observer for instance believed he could detect some rather uncertain physical signs with sufficient frequency to show, for instance, that a high proportion of old people were taking insufficient riboflavin, or another that children in substantial numbers were suffering from 'subclinical rickets'. The only answer to claims of that kind may be a rigidly controlled feeding test.

The Committee on Medical Aspects of Food Policy has approached this problem mainly through the development of a system of surveys used for those groups in the population which might be most susceptible to harm from suboptimal nutrition, combined with such general observations as the gain over the years in height and weight of schoolchildren, as compared with their predecessors in the same age groups, and a continuing watch on the range in quantity and quality of food taken.

I am not going into details on nutrition surveys because Dr Berry and Dr Darke have been closely concerned with the work and are far better able to describe it than I, but it illustrates the very different approach to nutrition in relation to public health which we must now use. We are watching the trend over a period in a group, rather than attempting to use clinical malnutrition in the individual as the index.

Every second year, as Chief Medical Officer of the Department of Education and Science, I am responsible for a report on the health of the schoolchild. Those reports go back for over 60 years to the first published by Sir George Newman and comment on the nutritional state of school-children has been a regular feature of them. That nutritional state has to be assessed by doctors undertaking routine examination of children, not using any standard of weight or height, but a clinical guess. Sixty years ago, and even 35 years ago, it was easy enough to point to children whose clinically observed nutritional state was certainly suboptimal as a result of their food intake being insufficient. Now it would be easier, using that method, to pick out children whose nutritional state was suboptimal because their intake of food was excessive and often ill chosen. Most of the children who are now recorded as malnourished are so because of some other physical condition and not from simple lack of food. That does not mean that the rest are all well nourished, but only that mild degrees of suboptimal nutrition do not lend themselves readily to clinical detection or accurate measurement. A few instances of specific clinically detectable vitamin deficiencies are found in young and old. Such cases are the result of particular individual social circumstances and are isolated, except that customs of some immigrant groups are such that their traditional feeding methods in the unaccustomed climatic conditions of this country are more likely than those of our own indigenous population to lead to lack of vitamin D. We may be confronted by unfamiliar problems if we seek to supplement their diet.

A related problem may exist among the increasing number of old or very old people in our population. One of the great uncertainties in this area is the significance of vitamin D intake in the aetiology of osteoporosis and so of the incidence of fractures, particularly of the radius and the femoral neck and particularly in women in later life. There is a plausible theoretical case for such an association. Nevertheless much of the liquid milk in the United States has been fortified with vitamin D for over 20 years and despite this the age specific death rates from falls in this older age group do not differ between the United States and Britain. Of course it may be that environmental conditions or systems of reportage render comparisons invalid, but this is an area in which further exploration is obviously needed and it is one of the easier examples of the kind of epidemiological study now needed in the nutritional field. It may well be that nothing less than a major controlled trial, using dietary supplementation, can provide the answer; but the cost of such a trial would be heavy and present investigation is directed rather towards seeking justification for such an effort.

The suggestion that subclinical vitamin D deficiency in children was far more widespread than had been recognised was investigated recently by a special panel of the Committee on Medical Aspects of Food Policy. The biochemical and radiological evidence of so-called subclinical rickets which was produced failed to convince the Panel, which did not recommend any change in our system of fortification of foods for infants with vitamin D, even though the amounts of vitamin D in the diets of many children were low.

This is another illustration of the impossibility of assessing the nutritional state through mere record of the dietary intake. The National Food Survey gives information about consumption, classified by various income and family groupings. These show that apart from vitamin D the poorest group of larger families with young children on average has intakes which should be sufficient to maintain health, but this lowest 7% of families may not be fairly represented by averages. The intake of the individual family will be affected not only by the money actually expended on food but by the skill with which it is expended. That may well mean that, qualitatively or quantitatively or both, those of the families in this group, perhaps with mothers such as those called in a 20-year-old investigation in Newcastle 'non-copers', may fall below the desirable levels. After all less than £14 a week income does not give much margin for mismanagement of a household with children.

There are other factors too which may affect the nutritional state of the individual child. It may well be that the great reduction in communicable disease in childhood, which leaves us now with a mortality from the five principal childhood diseases in that group less than 1 % of what it was 40 years ago (and an incidence very substantially if not proportionally reduced), has also reduced the threat to the nutritional state of the child. The relationship between measles infection in early childhood in some parts of Africa and the subsequent occurrence of kwashiorkor is well known. Even the common infections of childhood which are not notifiable specific diseases may well be reduced in their duration and effect by the drugs available now. The frequency of admission of children to hospital has undoubtedly been greatly reduced and the amount of time spent in hospital even more so.

Mortality at all ages up to 15 has been reduced in the last 40 years; by seven-eighths at ages 1–4; by five-sixths at ages 5–9, by more than three-quarters at ages 10–14. Some part of this is almost certainly the result of improved nutrition and the rest by prevention or control of acute infections. The general nutritional state of children therefore both assists, and benefits from, the improved health record.

It is possible that we will soon be able to check intake more accurately, as a result of more refined methods of estimating vitamin D in blood, but that does not tell us what the minimum or the optimum should be. Even if we could define the minimum needed to prevent rickets or osteomalacia or any earlier preclinical stage we will have a long way to go before anything of that kind becomes a routine procedure usable on a large scale. Moreover, there may be variation in absorption as in gluten sensitive enteropathy. There is perhaps a parallel in some very old observations about the excretion of ascorbic acid (vitamin C) and the concept of saturation as necessary to health. A far lower level of intake of ascorbic acid than is needed for saturation is perfectly compatible with health; yet levels of intake far above those on which we can maintain what appears to be normal health are commonly put forward as desirable. Only three months ago a paragraph about influenza in a leading national newspaper advised sufferers to go to bed at once and take vitamin C. Last week there was a paper suggesting some effect on the common cold. It really is not for me to offer an answer, but we need a lot more evidence to provide any certainty.

In the 12 years during which I have been Chairman of the Committee on Medical Aspects of Food Policy we have been moving from attempts to extrapolate from information about intake to attempts to make assessments by clinical and laboratory methods in the field. We have had some studies of the use of supplements, particularly iron in flour and vitamin D in the infant diet. So far the results have merely posed yet further problems for elucidation. One trial of iron supplements produced little or no reduction in anaemia. Serum alkaline phosphatase has been shown to fluctuate independently of vitamin D.

Government policy of using a selective rather than an overall method of supporting nutrition in childhood has recently aroused fierce criticism amongst many people, but not from those with real understanding of the nutritional field. Whereas during rationing it was essential to ensure the right quality and quantity of certain foods, out of a limited total national supply, for the vulnerable younger age groups and expectant mothers; when all important foods are freely available, if they can be purchased, the great majority of the population do not need special arrangements for provision that they or their parents understand and are able to make. The real problem then becomes that of ensuring that selective arrangements for those with insufficient resources do maintain the necessary diet for their children. It has been said that changes should not be made without evidence, but the fact is that evidence can only be obtained by making changes. What we must do, as a preventive measure, is to watch closely those groups where an adverse effect would first manifest itself, if it were to occur at all, and be ready to identify and report any deterioration at once. The assessment is extremely difficult, because for over 30 years the trend in height and weight at the different ages of childhood has been upward. Obviously that trend will not continue at the same rate indefinitely, but it makes the identification of an adverse effect attributable to diet extremely difficult. It is fortunate that COMA set up the machinery by which such observations can be made, and perhaps the simple observations of height and weight made through the School Health Service will be as important as anything of a more sophisticated kind. Our policy must be to try to eliminate malnutrition, the result of want, as far as this can be achieved by central policy. The local application of that policy will depend upon the identification of groups with special needs. It will be the quality of any supplementation that will matter more than the mere provision of energy.

We have had ways of dealing with the special problems of children and of expectant mothers in general during the time of rationing. The problem of the future lies rather in finding ways of ensuring that a minority in need can have the necessary supplement.

At the other end of the age scale there is a different kind of problem. COMA's recently published report, 'A Nutrition Survey of the Elderly', shows that a small minority were not adequately nourished. The explanation was in most cases, but not in all, some other concurrent departure from normal health which produced malnutrition as a secondary consequence. It may be that the small group remaining without an identifiable cause is undernourished not because of poverty but because of inability to make the best use of funds available. The King Edward Fund in their study of the nutrition of a group of old people, and particularly in the follow-up to that study, showed that the physical condition of most was satisfactory for their ages, but again a minority had not a suitable diet and appeared not to care or not to be able to care. It may be that the inability to care led to the unsatisfactory diet, but if that is so, then our efforts have to be directed to attempting to prevent that occurrence. In a group such as described in the study of 'The Old and Cold in Islington', the competition between adequate heating and adequate food—the worst kind of competition in those circumstances—went the wrong way for health. The same factor may be present in another study which reported too many old and cold. But our services ought to aim at preventing that competition from occurring. It is not enough to stand aside and say that such people could feed themselves properly on what they have got—if they would. The fact seems to be that they just have not the ability to use what they have to best advantage and that means not that we are excused responsibility but that we have to find a different way to help. Such a detectable small group may be helped by a selective approach; the possibility that others had suboptimal nutrient intakes without demonstrable ill effects must remain.

The choice of food is not so simple now as 20 years ago. The development of a vast range of convenience foods and the competition between convenience and cost makes the family's choice both economically and nutritionally more difficult. There are also new foods coming into use. The so-called filled milks came into infant feeding, first in hospital use, then much more widely, and a difficult problem of quality had to be resolved. Behind it all lies the uncertainty about whether it is sufficient to ensure adequate quantities of the components of the diet that we already know to be necessary. There may be other components of a traditional diet that have an importance we have not yet ascertained. The question comes up urgently now with the new protein foods of vegetable or other origin. They may be chemically adequate in all the respects we know to be essential. Some may have the necessary amino acids and even the necessary amount of iron, but we do not know whether, after absorption, the same ingredients are available for metabolism as would be obtained from meat. At the same time these new proteins could be a valuable source of additional protein, even if it were not biologically equivalent to meat. As dietary supplements they could be shown to have increasing importance in the future, provided they are not used as complete substitutes for meat by the socioeconomic groups that perhaps have the greatest need of them.

The production of substitute foods is not new. We have had our troubles in food hygiene with artificial cream in 1940 and again in the 1950s. What is new is that there are new ways of producing protein cheaply by means of unicellular organisms and these will need careful study from the aspects of health and nutrition, and also there are spun protein foods which appear to be sufficiently similar to meat for the consumer to accept them as such (irrespective of whether they are sold as such). The spun protein which has been marketed does not have the same amino acid pattern as meat (for which, in fairness, it is not marketed as a declared substitute) and it does not contain the same amounts of all the other nutrients that go with meat.

In principle, foods which are judged to be substitutes for other foods (irrespective of whether they are thus marketed) ought to be their nutritional equivalent. Nevertheless there may be practical limits to the extent to which this principle can be applied. Other countries, which are represented at this symposium, must have thought deeply over this problem and it will be of interest to learn their attitudes. On the good side, let it be said that in a time of world meat shortage and with food prices such as we are experiencing, other sources of protein used as well as meat may have a social and economic value in facilitating adjustments to new dietary patterns providing that they are without nutritional harm. Here, and in sorrow rather than in criticism, I must point to the substantial differences in the amounts recommended by different authorities not only of protein but of other nutrients also, which make it difficult for the administrator, medical or not, the politician or the public to judge.

Malnutrition, as a cause of ill health and disease may well be still declining in this country despite our inability to demonstrate unequivocally that this is so, but we know that in the public health field the least well-to-do socioeconomic groups have far worse mortality and morbidity statistics and these may be the effect rather than the cause of the low economic status. It is in this group that most of those whose nutritional state is marginal or worse will be found and it is a reasonable hypothesis that that fact makes a substantial contribution to the poorer health record to which their vital statistics testify. We are beginning the investigation of the problem of intervention in such a situation, an investigation that must be properly planned as an epidemiological exercise with adequate control. While that remains the main public health problem in nutritional science in Britain, another and relatively newly recognised problem emerges.

There are other disturbances of health which are the by-product of affluence. Obesity and perhaps physical inactivity are the most obvious of these. Both are conditions which can be remedied by personal adjustment of patterns of living and it would seem easy to say that the individual, here at least, can be left to look after himself. So he can, provided we can tell him how to do it, and within this particular problem there is that of the relationship of diet to the pathogenesis of atherosclerosis. At the present time one of the panels of COMA has been engaged for nearly two years in attempting to produce an agreed review of this subject. Some influential medical authorities, official and non-official, in other countries, especially in the United States and Sweden, have ventured on advice about causal relationships and there is some new Finnish evidence now. It does not seem that generally acceptable conclusions can yet be reached—a view recently given also by a committee of the New Zealand Heart Foundation. About the only firm ground seems to be that overweight and under-exercise are both disadvantageous. I have been told that the solution for the sedentary is a dog requiring half an hour's brisk walk daily—but then you have to be able to afford the dog and his house room. The formula seems a highly selective one to me.

Two months ago I was attending the Executive Board of the World Health Organization in Geneva. As always I was reminded at every turn of the comparatively trifling nature of our problems. We are seeking to identify a small minority of our young and old who have marginal states of defective nutrition—and so we should for most of us have more than enough. But in Africa and Asia at this moment there are literally hundreds of millions who do not have the minimum nutrient intake for good health. At the Executive Board of WHO in January we were discussing the spread of schistosomiasis round one of the huge man-made lakes in Africa. The population had benefited greatly from the addition of large amounts of protein to their diets from fish now so plentiful in the lake. They migrated to the shore to get the food. The snails which are intermediate hosts of the schistosomes could be killed quite easily by chemicals, but the fish would die too. The people could have food *and* schistosomiasis and they opted for that rather than going short of fish. That is a salutary reminder to us here, but no comfort either to the old lady who is neither warm enough nor sufficiently fed, and is too confused to handle either difficulty as she would have done 10 years ago when her husband was alive. Nor does it help the mother who has neither the personal capacity nor the rightful share of an exiguous family income to feed properly her existing children, or herself, in the current pregnancy. Those are the people about whom we should be most concerned in Britain today.

I fear that these random observations do much less than justice to the opening session of your research conference. They may seem to record no more than the puzzlement of the public health doctor faced with such an array of information to be applied to his problems. I think the lesson I have derived from 12 years in the Chair of COMA, on which Sir Frank Young has been such an important influence, is that we must do more to find out what actually happens in the human body and be less certain of extrapolation from food surveys and recommended allowances however widely accepted. FAO/WHO committees have attempted to replace some of the more arbitrary definitions of individual requirements by a range rather than an individual figure. But at the end of the day we have to do what has been recently done by John Waterlow, Walter Holland, Bill Berry and Sylvia Darke, Norman Exton-Smith, Chris Nordin and a host of others looking at people to try and ascertain what really happens to them, in the knowledge that the relevant laboratory studies are also being undertaken here in Cambridge, and elsewhere, so that we may eventually have better methods of objective appraisal of nutritional states.

I hope you will all forgive this somewhat unsophisticated collection of odd impressions, but I am sure you will all know how difficult it is to develop the kind of conspectus of nutrition in relation to health that is really needed for the formulation of policy now. May I say once more how much I personally am indebted to the effort that the group of experts who make up COMA and the large group who have contributed to the work of its panels have made with, I fear, all too little acknowledgment. I doubt if any other country has had more help of this kind.

I must make one last apology to the countries outside the British Isles. Hundreds of millions of people in other countries would be glad to have only the small problems I have discussed.

CHAPTER 2

Obesity—a problem in a changing world

W. J. H. BUTTERFIELD

Vice-Chancellor, University of Nottingham

My interest in the present subject really began in 1962 in Bedford during the diabetic survey I and my Department undertook there. We left our laboratories to study diabetes in the community believing that this condition might be attributable to underlying factors such as alterations in SH metabolism, probably on the surface of the mitrochondria, which we thought might explain our findings of elevated pyruvate levels in diabetes. But at Bedford we soon realised that just being overweight was probably more important than SH metabolism as a cause. Indeed, there was in Bedford in 1962 a reaffirmation, but in a reverse fashion, of what Bouchardat appreciated 92 years before during the siege of Paris, when he observed that losing weight alleviated all his diabetic patients in that city of hungry people.

THE COMPLICATIONS OF OBESITY

Obese patients have, until comparatively recently, been Cinderellas as far as clinical investigation has beeen concerned. In many ways, the diagnosis is self made and therefore subject to fashion. In view of the growing interest at present in self inflicted diseases, I must begin by pointing out that physicians are becoming more and more conscious of the many complications of obesity in addition to diabetes.

Does the extent of obesity influence the development of the different complications? One set of data amplifies this last point, namely, the relationship between the percentage over ideal bodyweight and the risk of diabetes. Research among US Government workers published by the US Public Health Service shows that for people under ideal bodyweight, the prevalence of diabetes, recognised by blood glucose measurements, was 0·7%, but this rose to 2% for those 20% overweight and to 10% for those 50% overweight.

These findings resemble the prevalence of overweight and of diabetes observed in various countries in the study led by Dr Kelly West from the USA. The population in Pakistan are on average less than the so-called ideal bodyweight in America and, interestingly enough, that nation has

13

14 W. J. H. BUTTERFIELD

less than 1 % of diabetics in surveys conducted there. At the other extreme, in the United States of America far more adults and young people are overweight and so is the prevalence of diabetes. Those who make international comparisons of the prevalences of diabetes are becoming suspicious that the apparent differences between countries are more closely related to the extent of obesity in the population than to any racial differences between the groups. Of course, there are exceptions: there are some exceptionally high prevalence rates in certain ethnic groups. But as far as I am aware, for all groups studied so far, being overweight is more important than any other factor in precipitating diabetes. It is time that similar correlative studies were made on a world wide basis for other complications of obesity.

THE DEFINITION OF OBESITY

If we are going to study obesity, we need to establish diagnostic criteria for it. Even if there is still not complete unanimity of world wide opinion about the diagnostic levels of blood sugar for diabetes, the WHO Expert Committee, to which I belong, made a try in 1964 (WHO, 1965), so there is no reason to evade the question of the definition of obesity. What should one take as being diagnostic of obesity? Fatfold thickness? Or some percentage in excess of the 'ideal' bodyweight? How should we attack this problem? One approach is as follows.

If we examine the relationship between morbidity from sudden death seen in groups of people of different degrees of overweight in the Framingham Heart Study in the United States of America, we find that there was, among men aged 30 to 59, a considerably increased mortality ratio for those whose weight was in excess of 119% of the 'ideal bodyweight'. In other words, being 20% overweight was associated with an increase in mortality.

However, this is admittedly a rather arbitrary definition of obesity and derived from a single age group.

Another approach would be to consider mortality generally, and with this in mind, and in an effort to exclude the variable of height, Seltzer used a form of the ponderal index (PI)—the patient's height in inches divided by the cube root of the weight, in pounds—as a basis for comparative studies of mortality (Seltzer, 1966). He observed that there is a relationship between excess mortality and decreasing ponderal index (that is to say, increasing obesity); thin people in the study with ponderal indices over 13 all had uniformly low mortality rates. I propose we accept his results as showing a possible inflection upwards of mortality at PI of 12·5 and a definite one at a PI of 12.

From these proposals, one deduces that to be of a PI greater than 12·5 is safe and to be of a PI less than 12 means one has a perceptible risk of increased mortality.

There are objections to these suggestions. For example, the ponderal index does not correlate very well with fatfold thickness, anyway not as well as does Quetelet's index, weight/height^2. The sort of difficulties that Seltzer's results bring to us may be demonstrated by setting out a table of heights with safe, borderline and dangerous weights based on the suggestions that a PI over 12·5 is safe and under 12·0 dangerous (*see* Table 1).

TABLE 1

SUGGESTIONS ABOUT SAFE AND DANGEROUS WEIGHTS

(Based on US Ponderal Index/Mortality Data)

Height ft in	Safe? PI 12·5 stone lb		Borderline? PI 12·0 stone lb		Dangerous?
6 2	14	11	16	11	
6 0	13	10	15	7	
5 10	12	8	14	2	
5 8	11	7	13	0	
5 6	10	8	11	12	
5 4	9	8	10	11	
5 2	8	10	9	12	
5 0	7	12	8	13	
4 10	7	1	8	0	
4 8	6	6	7	3	
4 6	5	10	6	7	

NB *See* text for interpretation.

If people look at this table, they tend to be unconcerned if they are tall and very concerned about their weights if they are short. Clearly there are difficulties about the sampling involved in this American study: we do not know how closely it matches the national population. Furthermore, it would not be easy to substantiate the two PI thresholds I have chosen, although I think two such points, safe and dangerous with an intermediate borderline range, have advantages over the blunter suggestion earlier, that weights in excess of 120% of the so-called ideal bodyweight are dangerous. There is also the point that these thresholds were based on mortality whereas it would be better to use morbidity as the basis for assessing dangerous weights.

One useful step would be to compare the figures in Table 1 with a random sample of the British population because this might give an indication of the prevalence of dangerous obesity as defined through ponderal indices. Furthermore, until we have a study of the heights and weights of a *random* sample of our population, we cannot say if there is a bimodal or continuous distribution of any index. In addition, there is a suspicion that the nation's physique is changing as a result of alterations in our cultural and economic backgrounds, our nutrition and indeed medical facilities. For example, presumably one reason young people today look like giants to the majority of old people is due to their having been protected by the antibiotic revolution from sharing nutrients with infective agents! As a result their growth curves have not had any interruptions due to infectious complications of the usual childhood illnesses.

There are conflicting views about whether the nation is getting more obese. Everyone I speak to tends to believe this and it seems supported by the fact that 20% of the population sampled in a recent survey admitted they had tried to lose weight during the preceding year through self diagnosing obesity. Were they right?

It has been pointed out by Mr David Donald of the Standard Life Assurance Company, that for those seeking insurance, the average weight for height has not changed. Of course, insurance groups are a highly selected part of the population and probably represent a class where physique has changed less, for example, than among the poorer classes where money has become available for food and where the ravages of infection have been reduced.

My own view, and I have expressed this elsewhere and repeatedly, is that we desperately need, in the United Kingdom, a national health survey of a randomly selected sample of about 10 000 people, to include heights and weights. I am chagrined that in the USA, where they do not have a National Health Service, they have had important baseline data about the nation's health from a national survey for over ten years, whereas we have had our health service but no such baseline to assess either our problems and priorities, or our health progress! As an aside, may I hereby give notice that I shall continue to lobby even more forcibly for a national health survey after April 1st 1974!

In the absence of such random sampling, one asks is there any possibility of constructing tables which might provide more reliable information about British physique than the widely used US Metropolitan Life Assurance tables? I was confronted with this problem several years ago when I was asked to recommend target weights for a scheme offering a computerised slimming diet to subscribers through a famous women's weekly newspaper published by IPC.

Constructing tables of current heights and weights would provide the opportunity to compare them with the approximations for dangerous weights in the foregoing table, and so derive a guide as to the prevalence of dangerous obesity for the last generation in society today. In attempting this, I was greatly helped by the work of one of my colleagues at Bedford in 1962, Dr Gillian Fowler (now Watkins) who recorded not only heights and weights but also other anthropological measurements on a random population sample. Her findings suggested that it might be possible to correlate body measurements with ponderal indices and these ideas were put to the test by my colleagues at IPC. By combining various sets of data available to them from the Women's Measurements and Sizes (Joint Clothing Council Survey, 1951), women's measurements on 2064 women by IPC Surveys Division in 1967, and the heights and weights reported by Montegriffo (1968) on 7301 males in 1964–66, and 'making creative use of the statistics', the IPC team produced the following estimates of mean weights and mean (M) plus 2 standard deviation (SD) weights for men and women of different ages (see Table 2).

TABLE 2

CALCULATED HEIGHTS AND WEIGHTS—MEN

(Derived from 3 British surveys 1951–67)

Height ft in	16–23 yr Mean stone lb	16–23 yr M + 2SD stone lb	30–44 yr Mean stone lb	30–44 yr M + 2SD stone lb	45 yr + Mean stone lb	45 yr + M + 2SD stone lb
6 2	12 6	15 3	13 5	16 7	13 3	16 12
6 0	11 11	14 6	12 10	15 10	13 0	16 2
5 10	11 2	13 9	12 2	15 0	12 6	15 5
5 8	10 8	12 12	11 7	14 3	11 11	14 9
5 6	10 0	12 3	10 13	13 7	11 3	13 13
5 4	9 5	11 7	10 5	12 10	10 9	13 2
5 2	8 12	10 12	9 11	12 0	10 0	12 6
5 0	8 4	10 2	9 2	11 4	9 6	11 10

Comparing the figures in Tables 1 and 2 it is immediately clear that very few of the taller men would be classified as dangerously overweight from my interpretation of Seltzer's results, but most short men would.

May we now consider the IPC data for women, which I suggest are reliable because out of over 30 000 women, we had very few complaints about the target weights we set them, which tended to be to get down to the mean weight for the individual height and age group: this certainly has not been so for previous tables. The IPC results are shown in Table 3.

Again, it is immediately apparent that very few of the tall women would be classified as overweight in Table 1, but the majority of short women would be! May I reiterate, we need a national health survey urgently and some sound prospective studies.

Meanwhile, one can only say that if the IPC trends were confirmed, as he gets older, modern man is getting grossly overweight, more so than modern woman, and this raises in my mind an interesting speculation about the health educational values of fashions!

TABLE 3

CALCULATED HEIGHTS AND WEIGHTS—WOMEN

(Derived from 3 British surveys 1951–67)

Height ft in		16–25 yr				30–44 yr				45 yr +			
		Mean stone lb		M + 2SD stone lb		Mean stone lb		M + 2SD stone lb		Mean stone lb		M + 2SD stone lb	
6	2	11	1	13	6	11	5	14	0	10	13	13	11
6	0	10	11	13	1	11	0	13	9	10	10	13	9
5	10	10	5	12	10	10	9	13	4	10	7	13	7
5	8	10	0	12	4	10	5	12	12	10	5	13	4
5	6	9	10	11	13	10	0	12	7	10	2	13	2
5	4	9	4	11	7	9	9	12	2	9	13	12	13
5	2	8	12	11	1	9	3	11	10	9	10	12	10
5	0	8	7	10	9	8	12	11	4	9	7	12	7
4	10	8	2	10	3	8	7	10	12	9	4	12	4
4	8	7	11	9	11	8	2	10	6	9	0	12	1
4	6	7	5	9	5	7	11	10	0	8	11	11	12

OBESE SUBJECTS—ENERGY BALANCE

Obesity is a result of overconsumption of energy against energy used. There have been various suggestions lately that as the human is only approximately 30% efficient it might be possible for obese persons to have a metabolic efficiency of more than 30%. This would explain the reports from apparently reliable sources that fat people consistently eat less than 1500 kcal (6·3 MJ) a day but fail to lose weight despite going about their daily business. I think all of us know of such cases: I certainly have a patient with dietetic training who makes such a claim and has produced records over several months to support her contention.

I have therefore been interested to receive information from Robert Bradfield and his colleagues (Bradfield, 1971; Bradfield et al., 1971; and Curtis and Bradfield, 1971) about their recent attempts to compare food consumption and energy expenditure in lean and obese American females, based on the analysis of closely kept records of eating and of energy expenditure, the latter being linked to estimates of pulse rate as reflections of oxygen expenditure. I need hardly add that other investigators have conducted similar studies before—I am thinking especially of studies of energy expenditure and food consumption of servicemen by Edholm and his colleagues and more recently oxygen and food consumption studies of soldiers under field conditions by Colonel Crowdy, to which I shall refer later.

However, the main points which result from the work of Bradfield and his colleagues worthy of mention here are these. First, the obese and lean females were roughly in energy balance as calculated, anyway to within about 5 % per day, suggesting that larger departures of metabolic efficiency from the normal range in obese subjects must be unusual. Second, the investigators found that some obese subjects had significant variations in their diet and their energy expenditure at the weekend compared to weekdays, obviously a very important point when designing laboratory studies of obesity. Third, the investigators did observe some differences in the very small amount of strenuous exercise taken each day, as expected more by lean (average weight 50 kg) than obese (74 kg) teenage girls.

This raises interesting points. We know now from the work of Barta and colleagues (Barta et al., 1968; Barta, 1969) that obese youngsters develop acidosis very quickly on exertion. This can be attributable to low muscle mass and the extra weight obese subjects have to move, though there may be other metabolic aspects of which we are unaware. The acidosis presumably induces breathlessness, making strenuous exercise potentially much more noticeable and unpleasant in obese subjects. Until they can develop a larger muscle mass, less prone to rely on anaerobiasis, to carry their excess weight, a vicious circle is established. So it may well be that the thresholds for so-called light, moderate and strenuous exercise in obese subjects are abnormally low. They may reasonably think that what makes them very breathless is heavy exertion, even though it is largely due to their muscle mass being so small that they get lacticacidaemia so much more easily than lean subjects. This point raises important questions about reliability of the pulse rate as a way of monitoring oxygen consumption in obese subjects. One is led inevitably to the conclusion that the subtler aspects of metabolic efficiency will not be resolved until investigators can make continuous measurements of oxygen consumption alongside continuous calorimetric measurements of heat output. We have of course the possibility of the former measurement through developments at the National Institute for Medical Research laboratories at Hampstead— Wolff's Portable Sampling Device—but future advances demand a major development in body calorimetry to get useful information about energy expended. It would be interesting to know if those Olympic swimmers do raise the temperature of the pool, though I doubt if they would appreciate the time they would have to wait in the water to get the baseline steady state readings! One wonders if flow calorimetry would help in this connection but even this will be complicated if the adipose tissue so lags the body that the core temperature rises sufficiently to initiate sweating. For we all know how easily plump people are brought to mopping their brows.

CARBOHYDRATE CONUNDRUMS

Although we are in doubt about the possibility that obese subjects have any overall alteration in metabolic efficiency we are gaining evidence that they certainly do have metabolic differences from normal subjects and those for carbohydrate handling are particularly well documented.

In the 1940s, Himsworth reported that when normal subjects had their .carbohydrate intake adjusted over periods of not less than three days, there were changes in the form of their glucose tolerance curve. On small carbohydrate intakes, normal subjects had a high glucose tolerance curve and when the tests were repeated after they had consumed more carbohydrate in their diet, the glucose tolerance curves got flatter. It is now widely recognised that as normal subjects eat more and more carbohydrate they adapt to this dietary change and although this may be related in part to enzyme adaptation, we appreciate from work in obese mice that the major tissue adaptation is an increase in the number of islet cells in the pancreas, permitting an increase in islet production of insulin.

We also now know that there are many metabolic differences related to carbohydrate and fat metabolism in obesity. Among the alterations Galton tabulated (Galton, 1968) one might note that the systemic level of glucose after an overnight fast is elevated in obese subjects, that the plasma insulin level at one hour of an oral glucose tolerance test is grossly elevated and the growth hormone levels, both basal and in response to insulin induced hypoglycaemia, are reduced. Furthermore, after obese subjects have lost weight, their growth hormone response to insulin is still less than in normal subjects. This last fact may be a very important clue about the setting of the hypothalamic mechanism associated with fasting and the release of growth hormone as a fat mobilising substance.

So far we have been discussing differences between systemic levels in normal weight persons and obese subjects. In fact, even more pronounced differences are discernible when one examines muscle metabolism as part of the metabolic symbiosis between the tissues. May I summarise first the findings in a report we have published recently. (Whichelow and Butterfield, 1971).

If one assesses fatness as fatfold thickness, there is an inverse relationship between obesity and how much glucose is taken up by the forearm muscles during the $2\frac{1}{2}$ hours following the administration of 50 g of glucose by mouth. The experimental data may be more meaningful if one takes the results and applies them on the assumption that the changes in the 30 kg muscle mass of an average person are comparable to the findings in the forearm. Such calculations show that an obese person takes up as little as 5 or even fewer of the total 50 g oral glucose load, into muscle, whereas a lean person may take some 40 g.

When we discovered this, the first thing that some of the plumper subjects among our laboratory colleagues said was, 'You have proved why I am fat, I have inherited muscles which are unable to use glucose. Professor John Yudkin is right. Providing I don't eat sugar, I won't have the excess glucose in my blood to be turned into adipose tissue'. And so on.

Unfortunately, other investigations show that obesity cannot be attributed simply to the inheritance of muscles which will not use glucose as a metabolic substrate. We find that, following several weeks' dieting, muscle glucose uptake in response to endogenous insulin rose towards the normal range. We now know that obese subjects do not have to lose much weight, as little as 5 or 6 lb, to get this order of improvement in the amount of glucose going into their forearm tissues. It is quite clear therefore that fat subjects are not fat because their muscles are refractory to glucose assimilation. And it should be added incidentally, they took up significantly larger amounts of glucose in the presence of quite high arterial levels of non-esterified fatty acids associated with the fasting which had brought about the weight loss, fasting which was maintained up until the morning of the second test.

Another extremely interesting finding is that, as people lose weight, their peripheral tissues become much more sensitive to insulin. This is shown by studies of four subjects before and after weight loss. Forearm uptake of immunoassayable (endogenous) insulin and of glucose was followed during oral glucose tolerance tests before and after dieting. When the four subjects lost weight their insulin uptake was increased, although the arterial insulin concentration was actually lower, and despite the reduced uptake of endogenous insulin, forearm glucose uptake was much greater. The mean results for the whole tests are shown in Table 4, from which it will be seen that there was a fourfold increase of insulin sensitivity after weight loss (Asmal *et al.*, 1971).

TABLE 4

EFFECTS OF WEIGHT LOSS ON PARAMETERS STUDIED

	Pre-therapy	*Post-therapy*
Arterial insulin concentration	104	82
Insulin uptake	104	45
Glucose uptake	540	1 030
Insulin sensitivity	5·3	23

We currently believe that weight loss can produce an increase in insulin sensitivity within seven days of the start of a low energy diet.

Obesity results from an imbalance between energy consumed and energy needs. Studies of the forearm give interesting data showing the effects of exercise on the one hand and, at the other extreme and in contrast, the effects of bed rest.

First, studies of exercise. It is possible to set up the forearm technique used in the previous studies and compare the uptake of glucose in one arm at rest with the contralateral arm doing exercise. Very light exercise, squeezing an unattached sphygmomanometer bulb once every ten seconds during the $2\frac{1}{2}$ hours of an oral glucose tolerance test, had a conspicuous roughly threefold effect on the response to the endogenous insulin secreted into the general circulation, compared to the uptake on the resting side. Other investigations have shown that this effect is *not* attributable to change of insulin sensitivity but is due to the increased amount of insulin filtered into the exercising muscles. (Garratt *et al.*, 1972). It is an interesting finding that if similar amounts of sugar went into all the muscles after meals, more than 50 g of glucose would be taken up there during the $2\frac{1}{2}$ hours following the oral administration of 50 g of glucose. Obviously, important regulatory mechanisms must be coming into action when exercise is taken after food and future research will probably reveal how important the hypothalamus is in this regulatory activity: the well recognised growth hormone released following exercise in diabetics may be a reflection of the breakdown of the normal servomechanism in patients with this disease.

By contrast when subjects rest in bed there is a change in insulin sensitivity of the forearm tissues; this has been reported by Lipman and his colleagues (Lipman *et al.*, 1972) who have shown that, if insulin is perfused into the brachial artery, the uptake of glucose is reduced after a week's bed rest. Thus, when patients are kept in bed their peripheral tissues become less insulin sensitive, consequently they need more endogenous insulin to dispose of a standard carbohydrate load in bed than when they are up and about: exactly how this jibes with the old adage—'feed a cold and starve a fever'—depends on whether you take to your bed with a cold. But one should certainly 'starve' if a fever takes one to bed, especially if one has impaired or suspect beta cell function, as in old age, or with a strong family history of diabetes!

I have been considering the results of investigations of an isolated part of the body, the forearm, representing muscles as part of the symbiosis in the body between the tissues. It is clear that as subjects become more obese less glucose moves into the muscle and that the muscles themselves become less insulin responsive. Where does the glucose go? Presumably into adipose tissue either in the abdomen or in the periphery. There is evidence both from *in vitro* and *in vivo* studies, that adipose tissue is less insulin sensitive than the muscle in lean circumstances, but it is possible that muscles in obese subjects have an insulin sensitivity comparable to adipose tissue so bringing the body towards a state of equilibrium in this respect. As we have shown that in the obese subject the muscle tissue insulin sensitivity is reduced to a quarter, it clearly needs more insulin to dispose of the glucose load, whether it goes into muscle or adipose tissue.

This contention is in complete harmony with the findings of Nikkilä and his colleagues who have been able, by isotopic dilution techniques, to assess the amount of insulin secreted through the liver into the systemic circulation following the stimulus of an oral glucose load. I should make it clear that it is not yet possible to measure in the intact man the actual amount of insulin released into the pancreatic vein. But a recent report by Nikkilä and Taskinen (1971) indicates how much more insulin has to be secreted into the general circulation in obese subjects to dispose of their blood sugar than obtains in non-obese subjects and, of course, as you would expect, in diabetics who are unable to respond to the rise of blood sugar with an increase of insulin released from the beta cells.

From all these results it is not surprising that when laboratory animals are given sufficient food to become overweight and subsequently killed, one finds in them larger numbers of beta cells in bigger islets than in non-obese animals.

It must be pointed out that all these measurements do not, of themselves, provide a full explanation of Himsworth's original findings to which I drew attention. The only conclusion we can make, and it is one that is acceptable today, is that with the increase in carbohydrate feeding there is a concomitant increase in insulin release which, in the short term, assists in the disposal of the oral glucose load in the mesenteric adipose tissue and the liver. Only in this way would it be possible to explain the lowering of the systemic glucose tolerance curve which Himsworth reported; changes in muscle uptake would be in the wrong direction.

But, before leaving this topic, I should perhaps re-emphasise the way in which obesity increases the demand for insulin to dispose of ingested carbohydrate, which probably explains the prevalence of diabetes with obesity.

THE ADIPOCYTES IN OBESITY—INCREASES IN SIZE AND IN NUMBERS

Obesity is due to excess energy laid down as fat in adipose tissue. The presence of excess lipid is reflected in the plasma too: obesity has been reported as associated not only with elevated levels of endogenous insulin, but also cholesterol, triglyceride and free fatty acids, and recent evidence shows a correlation between excess weight and glycerol levels.

An association has also been recognised by Abrams and other colleagues of my department at Guy's Hospital, London (Abrams *et al.*, 1969), between fasting plasma triglyceride levels and subsequent glucose tolerance: the higher the triglycerides, the higher the oral glucose tolerance test proved to be. Exactly how the relationship is brought about is not clear. Presumably elevated triglycerides are a reflection of a fat-laden insulin insensitive liver, as evidenced by the plasma insulin levels being raised so that the alteration in the glucose tolerance curve shows first that the liver is not sufficiently insulin sensitive to accept glucose from the portal circulation, and as the muscles are also insulin insensitive, the slow fall of the glucose level may reflect the slow disposal of sugar into relatively avascular adipose storage sites. Eventually the blood glucose falls back to the fasting level in these cases: that it takes longer is due to the changes I am suggesting in tissue symbiosis.

As fat is laid down, interest has centred on whether the adipocytes increase in number as well as in size. As far as the diabetic complication is concerned, this is of some interest because the available evidence suggests that insulin insensitivity of adipocytes is a reflection of their increased size. (Berchtold *et al.*, 1972; Stern *et al.*, 1972).

It is, I think, more difficult to answer this question than one might gather from reading the literature. Measuring the size and number of body adipocytes is not yet a very accurate procedure. Estimates tend to be based on relatively small biopsies of subcutaneous fat and enzyme treatment to break up the cell structure, from which calculations of cell size are made. The body fat content is then judged by estimates of total cell mass, using isotope dilution techniques. Another difficult assumption is that lipid is in adipocytes, whereas we know that it is also present in muscle, kidney and liver too. These sorts of problems explain the wide discrepancies between the estimates given for the numbers of adipocytes in man.

However, there is evidence based on standard measurements of adipocytes from three body sites, and using the same techniques in persons of various degrees of obesity before and after weight reduction. Per Björntorp and Lars Sjöström (Björntorp and Sjöström, 1971) have published good evidence that obesity is associated partly with increasing numbers of adipocytes, as well as increasing size. Furthermore, after weight reduction, the number of adipocytes did not fall proportionately.

This is important because it may explain the well known tendency of fat people to put on weight again after dieting, an experience so galling to those who successfully lose weight. Because, if the adipocytes only shrink, they become more insulin sensitive. Consequently, any overfeeding after slimming will make them highly susceptible to assimilate glucose. Perhaps the proper dietary advice to those who already have large numbers of adipocytes is to lose weight by any acceptable low energy diet, and to keep slim in our mechanised supermarket societies by avoiding excessive carbohydrate when you are slim!

Another interesting point is whether, by total fasting, one uses adipocyte protein and nucleic acids for body 'repair economy' as well as the lipid for energy. Do adipocyte numbers fall after total fasting? If so, lowering energy intake simply by restricting, say, carbohydrates or fat may leave the subject susceptible to a rapid weight gain later, by the mechanism I have suggested.

Björntorp and Sjöström have suggested that their data imply that there may be two sorts of obesity, that due to increased numbers of adipocytes (? in childhood), and that due to increased adipocyte size without material changes in the total numbers, but this is by no means proved.

There is some evidence in favour of their hypothesis from the work of Horton and his colleagues, who studied volunteer prisoners in Vermont and by dietary manipulation put the patients' weights up by 20 lb or more. (Sims *et al.*, 1969). The photographs published by the authors show how much of the adipose tissue was in the abdomen. Their biochemical studies showed the expected rises of blood cholesterol, triglyceride and free fatty acids, of insulin and the insulin glucose ratio. They also observed the well recognised deterioration of intravenous glucose tolerance and of greater growth hormone response to insulin. They observed a fall in total plasma ultrafiltrable cortisol, and a rise of cortisol production per kg. But they could find no evidence of increased numbers of adipocytes—in other words, their subjects expanded their adipocytes, but did not make new ones.

We see therefore that not only is there an interesting conundrum about the stimulus for multiplication of beta cells to make insulin, but also about the stimulus for multiplication of adipocytes to store the glucose the insulin is needed for: I shall be returning to this intriguing question later. But my colleague, T. E. Hanley, has been discussing this question of adipose mass, and the possibility that it is self regulating, for years.

Meanwhile, it is important to realise that, while we may be uncertain about these factors, there is evidence supporting the concept of fat mobilising substances which release lipid from adipocytes. There has been considerable discussion about this since Kekwick, Chalmers and Pawan described a fat mobilising substance they had detected by *in vitro* assay methods in the urine of fasting subjects. However, although the elusive substances have not yet been identified chemically, Curtis Prior has reported convincing evidence for the existence of a substance or substances affecting fat mobilisation. (Curtis Prior, 1973).

Another important aspect of metabolic significance is the question of uncoupling energy metabolism in such a way that the efficiency of thermogenesis is changed, so altering the usual relationships between excess energy consumed and the deposition of fat. Although there may be a gut regulator of energy absorbed, to which I shall also refer later, there is intriguing evidence from Derek Miller that some people can overeat without gaining weight. An explanation advanced for this phenomenon is that thermogenesis could account for the failure to gain weight unless food was consumed in two large meals a day in normal people.†

One suggestion for this metabolic inefficiency in normal subjects, by Stock and Stirling (*see* Cowling, 1972), is the ready availability of the enzyme alpha-glycerophosphate oxidase, permitting them to convert alpha-glycerophosphate away from being available for triglyceride synthesis and storage, and leaving fatty acyl coenzyme A, from free fatty acids, free for oxidation and heat production instead. If subjects were short of alpha-glycerophosphate oxidase, they would tend to synthesise triglycerides and become obese, and perhaps eating large meals overloads the enzyme and so results in the weight gain observed.

Once subjects have gained weight, certain other subtle effects have been noted, which may be relevant to the higher risks of death from coronary heart disease reported for overweight persons. Mahler has overfed students, one of whom noted a surprising deterioration in his athletic performance while he was obese, and a surprising delay in regaining his earlier time over middle distances on the running track. It is unlikely that a switch to fat metabolism by muscles would account for this. It can be argued that free fatty acids are much more efficient than glucose as a substrate for muscle: the extraction rate is 30% or more for each passage of the blood, as against less than 10% for glucose. Much more likely is the reduction in the lumen of the main arteries, in support of which are the reduced effective liver blood flows in obesity as reflected by prolonged BSP (bromsulphthalein) retention, and markedly reduced glomerular filtration rate as well as the personal observation that obese subjects, whom it may be remarked again easily become acidotic on exercise, also tend to have small and inconspicuous arteries: the difficulties with blood sampling in obese subjects is not only the adipose tissue, in my experience, but their sedentary state is usually also associated with smaller vessels, which being smaller are presumably more easily obstructed by athero-scelerosis or clot.

OBESITY AND THE CENTRAL NERVOUS SYSTEM (CNS)

Although the connections between carbohydrate consumption, insulin release and lipid deposition are becoming better understood, it should be noted that there must be a stimulus for the actual consumption of food to initiate the process of getting fat.

† It should be noted here that the long postprandial periods would be associated with release of growth hormone in the lean state; growth hormone is needed to multiply adipocytes in early infancy.

There is no doubt that if one injures parts of the hypothalamus of rats, either physically, with diathermy or simple traumatic ablation, or chemically with gold preparations, the animals become hyperphagic and, if the food is available to them, obese. The exact relationships between the lateral hypothalamic nucleus and the dorsomedial nucleus are not clearly worked out for man, but there is the possibility as a result of a new suggestion by Blundell (1971) that we may come to think of the lateral hypothalmus as putting out signals for feeding and hoarding food, depending on the overall nutritional status of the subject, and of the ventromedial nucleus as putting out signals, under post-feeding conditions, which intercept the feeding process, but not necessarily the hoarding instinct. In other words, satiety may not affect hoarding instincts and their possible hormonal connections. This suggestion becomes particularly interesting to me in relation to food consumption by the human female, who has a special hoarding system during reproductive life in addition to her larder, the mammae. There is evidence that the ventromedial nucleus affects prolactin release, though the exact interrelations are not yet understood for man. I am now trying to collect data about whether fasting or appetite supressants affect prolactin levels.

Apart from Blundell's intriguing suggestions about the interaction of nutritional status and post-ingestional stimuli, Anand and his colleagues in Delhi have reported (Anand, 1971) that in the rhesus monkey stimulation of the mesenteric afferent nerves evoked potentials in the region of the ventromedial satiety centre. When these afferents were stimulated after raising the blood level of the brain's main energy substrate, glucose, the evoked signals—to stop eating—were potentiated. Here we see a possible chain of events between brain glucose consumption falling, desensitising the ventromedial nucleus so that the feeding and hoarding signals from the lateral nucleus possibly originating from the 'hunger contractions' of the empty gut, create appetite, which in our society usually results in food consumption, rise of blood glucose which on the one hand causes endogenous insulin release and, perhaps associated with the latter, restores the function of the ventromedial nucleus, which cuts out the urge to feed, though not necessarily to hoard! The release of endogenous insulin can lead on, in appropriate circumstances, to the deposition of excess energy as lipid, both generally and in the adipocytes. And as the lipid deposition increases, so some tissues become less insulin sensitive—and less glucose enters the cells.

We have reported (Butterfield *et al.*, 1966) previously evidence which I still contend indicates that the CNS is insulin sensitive. I personally believe it quite likely that, with increasing obesity, there is diminishing uptake of glucose by the satiety centre in just the same way as occurs in the muscle in the obese subject's forearm. This slow glucose uptake would explain the observation, which I frequently make socially, that fat people eat very quickly, as though by forcing in the food, they push up their usually flat blood glucose level and so switch on the ventromedial satiety centre. It would also explain the loss of appetite after a few days rigorous dieting, when, I suspect, the satiety centre takes up glucose more easily, in the same way as obtains, as I said earlier, for the peripheral muscle.

Before leaving the question of cell uptake of glucose, it is interesting that an appetite suppressant, fenfluramine, has a definite metabolic action on muscle glucose uptake. Margaret Whichelow and I showed a conspicuous increase in glucose uptake during the $2\frac{1}{2}$ hours following oral glucose administration in a forearm perfused with fenfluramine administered intra-arterially, compared to the contralateral control forearm (Butterfield and Whichelow, 1968), and this has since been confirmed *in vivo* in man by Turtle and his colleagues in Sydney using a slightly different forearm technique devised by K. Zierler at Johns Hopkins and, in animals *in vivo* by Duhault in Paris and, *in vitro*, in the rat.

If such a direct metabolic action were effective in the CNS, then one might expect fenfluramine to produce similar effects to that produced by glucose and it is intensely interesting to me that this is precisely what Amand finds: injection of fenfluramine into the rhesus monkey increases signals evoked from the ventromedial nucleus in a way entirely comparable to that produced by glucose: I cannot help suggesting, due to local cell glucose assimilation.

These points link with other important aspects of obesity related to the CNS. Many years ago, Sturkard and Koch studied the relationships between gastric contractions and self reports of hunger in 37 obese subjects and 37 non-obese individuals, and found that, whereas with normal subjects the report of hunger was coincident with gastric mobility on 71 % of occasions, in obese subjects it was coincident in only 47·6%: in other words, obese subjects misinterpreted other sensations as hunger (Sturkard, 1959; Sturkard and Koch, 1964). More recently Schachter and his colleagues have been following up this idea that obese subjects have abnormal somatic sensibility. They have shown in a taste test that obese subjects, unlike normal weight people, eat *more* food when their stomachs are full than when they are fasting. (Schachter, 1970). Either obese subjects' appetites were not affected by the afferent impulses from distension of their stomachs, or they lost the taste of food under these circumstances. In view of Sturkard's work, the former explanation seems more likely, suggesting that the satiety centre was insensitive to the levels of metabolic substrates in the circulation after feeding, and to the afferent impulses from the bowels.

The bowels and the mesenteric afferents may well have a much more important role in weight control than we recognise. It is a well known fact that, on a weight reducing diet, faeces are smaller and harder, and that, when overeating, faeces are much looser and bulkier, suggesting some regulation in absorption. This notion is in harmony with the observations of Professor J. N. Hunt at Guy's Hospital who some years ago instilled a liquid diet, or a filler, by stomach tube into students on a measured diet and found the liquid diet given under these circumstances, did not produce the expected weight gain. Perhaps one needs to relish one's food to stimulate insulin and growth hormone release and become anabolic! Again, in the other direction, Colonel Crowdy of the Royal Army Medical Corps has been able to keep soldiers working on surprisingly low energy diets, providing they ate what seemed the normal combat ration. There may be gut regulators affecting absorption, much more important in energy balance than we currently realise.

THE ORIGINS OF OBESITY—IN EARLY LIFE OR IN EMBRYO?

In the last ten years there has been widespread realisation among physicians that all too frequently we are asked to intervene far too late in pathological processes to be of much avail. Looking back at any list of complications of obesity shows that the medical profession must take an active role in helping modern western man adapt to the non-famine technological society in which he finds himself. To be obese in famine-prone circumstances was an advantage—it clearly is not today.

How early on in life must doctors be introducing this help, as health education, for obesity? June Lloyd avers that obese children become obese adults and in Leeds, Professor Smithells (Smithells, 1972) has produced some alarming information about the prospects for obesity in the next generation based on his experiences about overweight babies today.
He wrote:

'In our studies of nutrition in pregnancy, we examine the babies when they are six months old. Our ancient departmental baby scales have proved useless because they only weigh up to 20 lb. *This was a reasonable weight for a baby approaching his first birthday* (my italics), but our six month babies have left it far behind. This is partly a matter of post-natal nutrition, but it illustrates, as does brain growth, that important patterns of development are laid down astonishingly early in life.'

Such rapid growth would not be feasible in primitive breast feeding societies, and a good deal of this appalling picture must be due to baby foods and early weaning onto ordinary meals.

One of the pioneers in the field of thought about the effects of metabolic abnormalities during embryonic life on subsequent developments was the late Professor Joseph Hoet of Louvain University. He persistently urged young research workers interested in the genesis of diabetes to study events in the pregnant woman, and follow her offspring for abnormalities of carbohydrate metabolism. Since his death, his son, Dr J. J. Hoet, now working in Brussels, has maintained an active interest in this field. The Hoet school will undoubtedly be interested in the growing attention being paid to these topics.

The general relevance of these comments takes on even more serious aspects when one considers them in relation to the recent report by Brook at the Institute of Child Health in London (Brook, 1972). He has suggested that the adipose organ in man has a finite sensitive period during which the basic number of cells is determined, and he puts this as from approximately 30 weeks gestation to the age of about one year. He believes the earlier the obesity-inducing events during this sensitive period, the more severe their effects, and suggests that after one year of age, growth in numbers is 'resistant to adverse circumstances'. It is interesting that he produces evidence that, if there is a deficiency of growth hormone, the number of cells is statistically significantly reduced.

There are more new data to link with this. Hellerström has recently shown (in pregnant rats) that slight foetal hyperglycaemia, produced by a 5% increase in total energy intake during the last 5 days of the animal's 21 day pregnancy, caused the beta cells of the offspring, studied *in vitro*, to release significantly more insulin in response to glucose than was seen with control beta cells. We see, therefore, that the overfed pregnant woman may prepare her unborn infant for hyperinsulinism, lipid-genesis and a less satiable appetitite. Unlike the Spartans, cross mothers cannot put their crying offspring onto a mountain side for the night: they quell the cries with more food! (Hellerström, 1973).

Dörner and Mohnicke (1973) have studied the effects of temporary hyperinsulinaemia during the period of thalamic differentiation in male rats. They report that some of the animals developed spontaneous hyperglycaemia, decreased glucose tolerance, hypercholesterolaemia and obesity in the subsequent life of the animals. Hoet would feel fully vindicated with this indication that foetal hyperinsulinism—he would have attributed it to the maternal hyperglycaemia—can lead on to obesity and diabetes.

In a way these findings are helpful to those of us interested in health education today because it is probably a more practical proposition to explain all these ideas to today's expectant mothers and the babies' grandparents (Bolte and Gleiss, 1969) than to get the babies themselves to change their behaviour. Nor should it be forgotten that health education in these matters is becoming more and more the responsibility of our health visitors who, on top of training first as a nurse and then as a midwife, have a year's course to prepare them and equip them to visit people in their own homes with a view to encouraging healthier living—a challenging and rewarding profession! And since they are almost all trained midwives, they should understand what we are getting at.

CONCLUSIONS

If obesity has been a self-diagnosed condition, it is fast becoming a national scandal. There is plenty of interesting work to be done on what has been regarded as a Cinderella condition. Unlike geriatrics, that other medical Cinderella—though some would see these two subjects as the Ugly Sisters! —there is a lot we ought and could be doing about obesity now which would be appreciated greatly by our successors in the medical profession next century.

Clearly there is practical health education to be undertaken to stop the babies getting any fatter. Obviously we need to know much more about the factors which 'set' the appetite and hoarding centres in the hypothalamus in late gestation and early life. We urgently need to know what makes adipocytes multiply. There is evidence that growth hormone is important. Derek Miller tells me that butter and egg powder make weakling rats grow fat; Mme Raulin has reported experiments which suggest that the DNA–RNA content of epididymal fat pads in young rats is greatest if the fat in the diet is as unsaturated fatty acids (Raulin, 1969), and Hugh Sinclair has kindly referred me to Kazdova and Vrana (1970) who found that carbohydrate and intraperitoneal, but not subcutaneous, insulin increased the DNA and RNA content of adipose tissue. Clearly this whole subject urgently needs exploration, not least because the highest quality baby food sold in The Netherlands is very rich in unsaturated fatty acids! We also need to know how to make adipocytes atrophy completely for the sake of those currently obese!

Throughout the foregoing presentation, I hope it has been clear that there are strong hormonal and metabolic threads, such as linking populations of islet cells with insulin production. I have also tried to draw attention to new ideas in our metabolic considerations, changes in the size of cell populations—which is propitious when there is so much concern about the size of human populations. As the economists are reviewing the effects of excessive growth and discussing and writing about 'no growth' systems, so physicians, and even, strange thought, paediatricians and obstetricians, are being drawn into similar trends of thought, anyway as far as beta cells and adipocytes are concerned!

If I have managed somehow to interest and stimulate just one or two able young investigators and educationalists to devote some of their talents and energies to this field of obesity, all my struggles to cannulate deeply hidden brachial arteries and anticubital veins in fat forearms were not entirely in vain!

REFERENCES

Abrams, M. E., Jarrett, R. J., Keen, H., Boyns, D. R., and Crossley, J. N. (1969). *Br. med. J.*, **1**, 599.

Anand, B. K. (1971). *S. Afr. med. J. Suppl.* 12.

Asmal, A. C., Butterfield, W. J. H., Cox, B. D., Karamos, B. and Whichelow, M. J. (1971). *Postgrad. med. J. Suppl.* June, 407.

Barta, L. (1969). *Pädiat pädol,* **5,** 13.

Barta, L., Szöke, L. and Vandor-Szobotka. (1968). *Acta paediat. hung.,* **9,** 17.

Berchtold, P., Björntorp, P. and Gustafson, A. (1972). *Acta med. scand.,* **191,** 35.

Björntorp, P. and Sjöström, L. (1971). *Metabolism,* **20,** 703.

Blundell, J. E. (1971). *S. Afr. med. J. Suppl.* 13.

Bolte, R. and Gleiss, J. (1969). *Kinderäztl Praxis,* **37,** 123.

Bradfield, R. B. (1971). *Am. J. clin. Nutr.,* **24,** 1148.

Bradfield, R. B., Paulos, J. and Grossman, L. (1971). *Am. J. clin. Nutr.,* **24,** 1482.

Brook, C. G. D. (1972). *Lancet,* **2,** 624.

Butterfield, W. J. H. and Whichelow, M. J. (1968). *Lancet,* **2,** 785.

Butterfield, W. J. H., Abrams, M. E., Sells, R. A., Sterky, G., Veall, N. and Whichelow, M. J. (1966). *Lancet,* **1,** 557.

Cowling, J. (1972). *New Scientist,* 6 July, 31.

Curtis, D. E. and Bradfield, R. B. (1971). *Am. J. clin. Nutr.,* **24,** 1410.

Curtis Prior, P. (1973). *Diabetologia,* April, **9,** 158.

Dörner and Mohnicke, A. (1973). To be published.

Galton, D. J. (1968). In *Clinical Endocrinology,* p. 721 edited by E. B. Ashwood and C. E. Cassidy, Grune and Stratton, New York.

Garratt, C. J., Butterfield, W. J. H., Abrams, M. E., Sterky, G. and Whichelow, M. J. (1972). *Metabolism,* **21,** 36.

Hellerström, H. (1973). *Abstracts of the Proceedings of the International Diabetes Federation* (to be published).

Joint Clothing Council Survey (1951). HMSO, London.

Kazdova, L. and Vrana, A. (1970). In *Proc. Int. Nutr. Congr.* p. 282. Excerpta med. Foundn, Amsterdam.

Lipman, R. L., Raskin, P., Love, T., Triebwasser, J., Lecocq, F. R. and Schnure, J. J. (1972). *Diabetes,* **21,** 101.

Montegriffo, V. M. E. (1968). *Ann. Hum. Genet.,* **31,** 389.

Nikkilä, E. A. and Taskinen, M. R. (1971). *Postgrad. med. J. Suppl.,* June, 412.

Raulin, J. (1969). In *Physiopathology of Adipose Tissue,* p. 76, edited by J. Vague. Excerpta med. Foundn., Amsterdam.

Schachter, S. (1970). In *The Psychopathology of Adolescence,* p. 197, Grune and Stratton, New York.

Seltzer, C. C. (1966). *New Engl. J. Med.,* **274,** 254.

Sims, E. A. H., Kelleher, P. E., Horton, E. S., Gluck, C. M., Goldman, R. F. and Rowe, D. L. (1969). In *Physiopathology of Adipose Tissue,* p. 78, edited by J. Vague, Excerpta med. Foundn., Amsterdam.

Smithells, R. W. (1972). *J. Health Educ.,* **31,** 40.

Stern, J., Batchelor, B. R., Hollander, N., Cohn, C. K. and Hirsch, J. (1972). *Lancet,* **2,** 948.

Sturkard, A. (1959). *Psychom. Med.,* **21,** 281.

Sturkard, A. and Koch, C. (1964). *Arch. Gen. Psychiat.,* **11,** 74.

Whichelow, M. J. and Butterfield, W. J. H. (1971). *Q. Jl. Med.,* **158,** 261.

WHO (1965). *Tech. Rep. Ser. Wld. Hlth. Org.,* No. 310.

CHAPTER 3

Fibre—is it a dietary requirement?

DENIS P. BURKITT

Medical Research Council External Staff, London

COMPOSITION, MISUNDERSTANDING AND NEGLECT

Food fibre has traditionally been defined as the part of the diet that is not destroyed by boiling in both dilute acid and dilute alkali. Not only is this a purely academic definition which bears little relationship to what happens to food in the gastrointestinal tract, but it takes no account of the pentosans which, though not digested by small bowel enzymes, are largely broken down by bacteria in the colon (Southgate and Durnin, 1970).

Because fibre has no nutritive value it has been classed as 'unavailable carbohydrate', although the lignin fraction is not in fact carbohydrate. Consequently it has been presumed to have no function in maintaining health, and has therefore been discarded as a food impurity. Although it has been the most neglected component of human diet its value has been appreciated by those concerned with animal husbandry.

THE EFFECTS OF FIBRE-DEPLETED FOODS ON THE GASTROINTESTINAL TRACT

Heaton (1973) has emphasised that part of the natural function of the gastrointestinal tract has been the removal of fibre from plant foods so as to render the contained starches and sugars available for absorption. In modern western society this function has been largely taken over by artificial food processing which removes most of the fibre before the food is consumed. This alters the normal physiological activity of the whole of the gastrointestinal tract.

The mouth
Effects on teeth
Acids produced by fermentation of sugars play a major role in causing dental decay. Soft starchy foods, particularly those composed of refined flour, hold the sugars and their fermented products in prolonged contact with the teeth and gums. Dental caries and periodontal disease result. Less refined diets are less cariogenic and foods requiring mastication have

a cleansing and abrasive and therefore protective action on the teeth and gums.

Effect of mastication
Coarse food requires more mastication than refined food and is consequently held for longer in the mouth before swallowing, as shown by McCance *et al.* (1953). As a result it reaches the stomach mixed with more saliva than does more quickly eaten refined food.

The stomach
Overconsumption
A high fibre content increases the bulk of a meal. Consequently the stomach is filled and appetite satisfied with less food and less energy than would be the case with concentrated refined foods which provide no bulk and so lead to overconsumption. Obesity, which is so closely linked with refined carbohydrate foods, may be due partly to overeating and partly to more complete absorption of the food ingested in the small bowel.

Delayed emptying
McCance *et al.* (1953) fed volunteers with meals consisting of equal weights of wholemeal and of white bread, and with radiological control showed that on average the former left the stomach one hour sooner than the latter. It is not known what pathological significance this may have, but there does appear to be a relationship between peptic ulcer and refined foods. Malhotra (1970) blames deficient mastication and mixing with saliva; Cleave (1962) blames protein stripping and Yudkin (1972) some action of sugar. Tovey (1972) obtained remission in peptic ulcer patients in India by adding rice bran to their diet.

The small intestine
Increased food absorption
There is some evidence that a greater proportion of nutrients, vitamins and minerals are absorbed from refined than from less processed foods. This could be an advantage or disadvantage according to the nutrition status of the community concerned.

The increased absorption from a low residue meal may in part be due to the fact that it takes longer to pass through the small intestine (McCance *et al.*, 1953).

When sugars and starches are consumed in a refined form they are absorbed from the small intestine much more rapidly than they would be if eaten in their natural state. Since the starches are turned to glucose after absorption this means that the pancreas may have to cope with a much more rapid intake of glucose to the bloodstream than that which naturally occurs. Cleave *et al.* (1969) postulate that this may be a fundamental cause of diabetes, a disease which is much more prevalent in communities eating a refined diet.

Reabsorption of bile acids and absorption of dietary cholesterol
More bile acids are reabsorbed from the terminal ileum on a refined than on an unrefined diet (Heaton, 1972). Since bile acids are formed from cholesterol there is less need for cholesterol to be used for this purpose if the bile acids are re-cycled.

More of the cholesterol eaten in food is believed to be absorbed on a low than on a high residue diet (Heaton, 1972). The fibre in the latter apparently binds the cholesterol and evacuates more of it in the faeces.

For both these reasons a low residue diet is believed to predispose to a build up of cholesterol.

Absorption of lithocholate
Lithocholate, a product of the breakdown of bile acids in the intestine, also tends with a low residue diet to be absorbed and returned to the liver. In contrast, on a high residue diet more of it is excreted in the stools. The absorbed lithocholate suppresses the breakdown of cholesterol into bile acids (Heaton, 1972).

For these reasons a fibre depleted diet may be an important cause of coronary heart disease. Trowell (1972*a*, *b*) has accumulated much evidence that relates low residue diets with this commonest killing disease in the western world.

Heaton (1972) believes that the build up of cholesterol relative to bile salts which keep bile cholesterol in solution, is an important cause of cholesterol gallstones. These, like coronary heart disease, are very common in economically developed countries and are rare in most less westernised communities.

The large intestine
Intestinal transit times
Numerous studies have indicated that the speed of passage of faeces through the large bowel is profoundly influenced by the fibre content of the diet. The effects of particularly high or low residue diets are seen in African villagers living on an almost totally unrefined diet who have been shown to pass 80% of ingested radio-opaque markers within 30–40 hours of swallowing, and astronauts fed on a fibre free diet who can go for a week or more without passing a motion (Winitz *et al.*, 1965). Between these extremes people in developing countries eating a mixed diet, and vegetarians in England, have intestinal transit times averaging about two days, and those on more refined normal western diets averaging more than three days, and often over four (Burkitt *et al.*, 1972).

Stool weights

While the fibre content of diet is inversely related to intestinal transit time it is directly related to stool bulk and weight. Rural populations in developing countries consuming unrefined foods usually pass over 300 g and not uncommonly over 500 g of stool a day. In contrast, the daily stool weights of those on British or North American diets average well under 150 g.

Stool consistency

The more rapidly passing large stools associated with high residue diets are characteristically soft and usually unformed, whereas those associated with low residue diets are firm and often faceted.

Intraluminal pressures

The muscles in the intestinal wall have to work much harder on a low than on a high residue diet in order to propel the small, firm faecal masses along the lumen of the colon. The strong muscular contractions required build up unnaturally high pressures in the lumen of the bowel. Soft bulky stools associated with high residue diets are propelled through the intestine much more easily, and intraluminal pressures are consequently markedly smaller (Painter, 1964, 1967).

Restoration of normal bowel function following replacement of fibre

Although bowel function can be shown to be related to the fibre content of food it might be argued that it is some other constituent of diet that is the important factor. The observation that the restoration of quite small amounts of cereal fibre, often no more than 2 g/day radically alters bowel behaviour (Painter *et al.*, 1972), suggests that dietary fibre is indeed a crucial factor. Fibre from cereals and legumes has been shown to be more effective than fibre in fruits and green vegetables in influencing bowel activity (Hoppert and Clark, 1945).

DISEASES OF THE LARGE BOWEL RELATED TO FAECAL ARREST

Constipation

A low residue diet is the most important cause of constipation (Jones, 1972). Over £6 million are spent annually in Great Britain on laxatives, which are taken regularly by an estimated 15 million people. The addition of fibre to the diet in the form of unprocessed bran would be a cheap and effective remedy.

Appendicitis

Even in the western world appendicitis was rare before the present century (Short, 1920). It is still rare in rural communities in developing countries but is becoming increasingly common amongst those who have adopted European types of food (Burkitt, 1971a). It is believed that the fundamental cause is obstruction to the lumen of the appendix either by a faecalith or by muscular contraction, both of which are related to low residue foods. Pressures build up behind the obstruction, and cause damage to the mucosal lining of the appendix which allows bacterial invasion. Diet also causes changes in bowel bacteria and this probably contributes to the development of appendicitis (Cleave et al., 1969).

Diverticular disease

This is the most common intestinal disease of the western world where it was rarely seen before the second quarter of the present century. It is still exceedingly rare in developing countries where most of the population live on high residue diets. It is believed to be caused by the high pressures produced in the bowel by low residue diets as described above. These pressures force the mucosa through the muscle layers of the intestine.

A high fibre diet is becoming increasingly recognised as the best treatment for the disease.

Benign and malignant tumours

Cancer of the large bowel is second only to lung tumours as a cause of death from cancer (Doll, 1969). Simple bowel tumours are probably present in about one in 5 of the adult population in Britain and North America (Arminski and McLean, 1964). Both these conditions are rare in developing countries.

It is now believed that the action of bacteria on normal bowel constituents may produce the substances responsible for bowel tumours (Aries et al., 1969; Hill et al., 1971). Any potential carcinogens so formed would, in the presence of the faecal arrest associated with low fibre diets, be held against the mucosal lining of the bowel for a prolonged time concentrated in a small faecal mass. Under these circumstances more tumours might be expected to develop than with a high residue diet when less carcinogens might be formed, and those which were formed would be diluted in a large faecal mass and pass more quickly through the colon and rectum (Burkitt, 1971b; Oettle, 1967).

DISEASES ASSOCIATED WITH RAISED INTRA-ABDOMINAL PRESSURES

As shown above the constipation consequent on a low residue diet causes raised intraluminal pressures in the colon. It also results in straining at stool which causes unnaturally raised intra-abdominal pressures. These pressures are transmitted to the veins of the lower limbs and pelvis and may be an important cause of varicose veins and haemorrhoids (Burkitt, 1972a). It seems likely that raised intra-abdominal pressures also contribute to the cause of hiatus hernia (Burkitt, 1972b).

All these conditions are rare in communities living on high residue diets.

CONCLUSION

There is good evidence that fibre-depleted diets cause pathological effects not only in the gastro-intestinal tract, but also in other structures including the arteries, lower limb veins and gall bladder. There is no evidence that the restoration to our diet of fibre in the amounts that would seem necessary to combat these diseases could do any harm and it would appear to be a case of 'heads I win and tails I don't lose'. With odds of this nature the only logical step seems to be an endeavour as individuals and as members of a community to restore the cereal fibre which has been removed from our food.

The hypothesis formulated in this paper was largely inspired by the work of Captain T. L. Cleave whose original concept of a 'Saccharine Disease' deserves careful consideration by all those concerned with diet and disease.

REFERENCES

Aries, V., Crowther, J. S., Drasar, B. S., Hill, M. J. and Williams, R. E. O. (1969). *J. Br. Soc. Gastroenterol.*, **10**, 334.

Arminski, T. C. and McLean, D. W. (1964). *Dis. Colon Rectum*, **7**, 249.

Burkitt, D. P. (1971a). *Br. J. Surg.*, **58**, 695.

Burkitt, D. P. (1971b). *Cancer*, **28**, 3.

Burkitt, D. P. (1972a). *Br. med. J.*, **2**, 556.

Burkitt, D. P. (1972b). 'Geographical Pathology Related to Diet'. *The Medical Annual*, John Wright and Sons Ltd, Bristol.

Burkitt, D. P., Walker, A. R. P. and Painter, N. S. (1972). *Lancet*, **2**, 1408.

Cleave, T. L. (1962). *Peptic Ulcer*, John Wright and Sons Ltd, Bristol.

Cleave, T. L., Campbell, G. D. and Painter, N. S. (1969). *Diabetes, Coronary Thrombosis and the Saccharine Disease*, 2nd ed., John Wright and Sons Ltd, Bristol.

Doll, R. (1969). *Br. J. Cancer*, **23**, 1.

Heaton, K. W. (1972). *Bile Salts in Health and Disease*, Churchill Livingstone, Edinburgh.

Heaton, K. W. (1973). Personal communication.

Hill, M. J., Crowther, J. S., Drasar, B. S., Hawksworth, G., Aries, V. and Williams, R. E. O. (1971). *Lancet*, **1**, 95.

Hoppert, C. A. and Clark, A. J. (1945). *J. Am. diet. Ass.*, **21**, 157.

Jones, F. Avery (1972). 'Management of Constipation in Adults' in *Management of Constipation*, p. 97, edited by F. Avery Jones and E. W. Godding, Blackwell Scientific Publications, Oxford.

Malhotra, S. L. (1970). *Amer. J. dig. Dis.*, **15**, 489.

McCance, R. A., Prior, K. M. and Widdowson, E. M. (1953). *Br. J. Nutr.*, **7**, 98.

Oettle, A. G. (1967). 'Primary Neoplasms of the Alimentary Canal in Whites and Bantu of the Transvaal, 1949–1953. A Histopathological Series', in *Tumours of the Alimentary Tract in Africans*, National Cancer Institute Monograph 25. Bethesda, Maryland.

Painter, N. S. (1964). *Annals Roy. Coll. Surg. Eng.*, **34**, 98.

Painter, N. S. (1967). *Amer. J. dig. Dis.*, **12**, 222.

Painter, N. S., Almeida, A. Z. and Colebourne, K. W. (1972). *Br. med. J.*, **2**, 137.

Short, A. R. (1920). *Br. J. Surg.*, **8**, 171.

Southgate, D. A. T. and Durnin, J. V. G. A. (1970). *Br. J. Nutr.*, **24**, 517.

Tovey, F. (1972). *J. Christian med. Assoc. of India*, **47**, 312.

Trowell, H. (1972a). *Amer. J. clin. Nutr.*, **25**, 926.

Trowell, H. (1972b). *Eur. J. clin. biol. Research*, **17**, 345.

Winitz, M., Graft, J., Gallagher, H., Narkin, A. and Seedman, D. (1965). *Nature, Lond.*, **205**, 741.

Yudkin, J. (1972). *Pure, White and Deadly*, Davis-Poynter, London.

CHAPTER 4

The Common Market and food and nutrition in Britain

G. A. H. ELTON

Chief Scientific Adviser (Food),
Ministry of Agriculture, Fisheries and Food, London

The United Kingdom has been a member of the European Economic Community for three months, but the effects, if any, that joining will have on our diet are still extremely difficult to assess. Nutritionists are most interested in any changes which will occur in our energy and nutrient intakes, but these depend on changes in the amounts of the various foods we eat, which in turn depend on changes in supplies and relative prices and on the response of the consumer to these changes.

The most important reason for the uncertainty is that any changes directly attributable to entry will be spread over a long period. Adoption of the Common Agricultural Policy, with its emphases on free movement of goods within the community, on common frontier tariffs for foodstuffs imported from outside the community, and on farmers getting a greater proportion of their return from the consumer than the taxpayer—all of which affect the availability and price of food—will not be complete for five years. And other legislative changes which could affect the composition of our food will come into operation only after detailed discussion between the member countries, so the results cannot easily be predicted.

During this time many other factors can arise to confuse matters. For example, during the past year, diverse factors entirely unconnected with our entry into Europe, such as the failure of grain harvests in Russia and China, droughts in Australasia, shortages of fish in the North Atlantic and near Peru, and a rising world demand for beef, have caused large increases in the prices of wheat, fish and meat. Other factors which could affect food consumption patterns in Britain, but may be only marginally connected with EEC entry, include: (1) changes in people's disposable income, or the proportion they are willing to spend on food; (2) introduction of new products by food processors, because of technological innovations or to satisfy the demands of a more widely travelled or immigrant population; (3) changes in the size, age structure, regional distribution or physical activity of the population; and (4) strong medical or nutritional advice for or against consumption of certain foods.

The Government have, however, several very effective continuing surveys for monitoring whatever changes do occur. The three major ones are described briefly, and the trends they have shown projected to suggest what consumption patterns might have occurred had Britain not joined the EEC. Finally, comparisons with consumption trends in the original EEC countries will be used to indicate what changes could result from Britain's entry.

FAMILY EXPENDITURE SURVEY

The FES has been conducted by the Department of Employment continuously from 1957. For households of different family composition and income ranges including pensioners, and in different geographical areas (for example), it shows expenditure not only on food and alcoholic drink, but also on housing, fuel, light and power, tobacco, clothing and footwear, durable household goods, other goods, transport and vehicles, services, and miscellaneous items. Within each of these broad areas there are further subdivisions, 'food' being divided into 32 items including, for example, six different kinds of meat, as well as expenditure on meals bought away from the home. The FES is therefore a consistently reliable source of information on household expenditure in the United Kingdom, despite three drawbacks. First, there is evidence of underreporting of expenditure on items about which society tends to disapprove, such as alcohol and to a lesser extent sweets and ice cream; this would slightly raise the proportion of household income which appears to be spent on more staple foods. Secondly, the response rate to the interview and complicated questionnaire among the 11 000 randomly selected householders is only 70%. And thirdly, no account is given of the quantities of food purchased or of its nutritional value.

For the past 10 years, the proportion of our income which has been spent on food has steadily declined, from about 30% in 1962 to about 25% in 1971, while the proportion which has been spent on alcoholic drink has risen during the same time from 3·8% to 4·7%. There has in fact been a marked general trend away from more basic items towards 'luxury' items during this time for most sections of the population. It remains to be seen whether these trends continue during the next five years while the Common Agricultural Policy is being adopted.

No other country in Europe has such a comprehensive continuing survey, but some approximately comparable figures for the proportion of the national income which is spent on food and drink (Table 1) show that the United Kingdom has been in an average position. The proportions were higher in previous years.

TABLE 1

PERCENTAGE OF NATIONAL INCOME SPENT
ON FOOD AND DRINK IN THE UNITED
KINGDOM AND ORIGINAL EEC COUNTRIES
(1969)

West Germany	20
Netherlands	20
Luxembourg	22·5
Belgium	23
UK	25
France	25
Italy	32

CONSUMPTION LEVELS ESTIMATES

The CLE began before the Second World War, and show the total amount of foodstuffs available in the United Kingdom at a primary stage of distribution. They are calculated yearly by the Ministry of Agriculture, Fisheries and Food from information on the home production of food together with imports, less deductions for exports and non-food uses of the material. This survey can be matched in most developed countries, so the food available per head in the UK can be compared with that available in, say, the USA as well as the original members of the EEC. The Organisation for Economic Co-operation and Development (OECD) compiles these data and even allows a few nutritional comparisons, for information is also presented on the energy, protein and fat content of this food.

NATIONAL FOOD SURVEY

The NFS, undertaken by the Ministry of Agriculture, Fisheries and Food since the beginning of the Second World War, amplifies one aspect of the FES by providing much more detailed information on household consumption of and expenditure on food. This survey shows, for households of different family composition and income ranges, and in different geographical areas, the amounts of more than 130 different foodstuffs which are purchased (or obtained free) throughout the year. A nutritional interpretation is also provided: for each type of household, the amounts of energy, fat, carbohydrate, protein (including animal protein), calcium, iron, thiamin, riboflavin, nicotinic acid, and vitamins A, C and D in the diet are assessed both absolutely and in terms of the intakes recommended by the Department of Health and Social Security.

This survey is, like the FES, invaluable in providing breakdowns which are both truly national (allowing cross-sectional studies at any point in time) and continuous (allowing the study of time series); it also has limitations in that it cannot provide information on intakes by individuals or on foods which are outside the housewives' knowledge (such as alcohol, sweets, and certain aspects of meals purchased outside the home). Furthermore, the response rate among the 15 000 randomly selected households is little over 50%.

Further analyses are made, the most important to the present topic being 'price elasticities of demand'. These are mathematical expressions of the way in which price changes affect purchases of a food, either in isolation or in terms of other closely related foods. Thus, within known ranges a certain percentage increase in the price of beef would lead to an approximately predictable decline in the purchases of beef and transfer to purchases of other meats such as poultry.

No other country in Europe has such a comprehensive and regular survey.

The NFS provides such a wealth of information that it is central to Government plans for monitoring any changes which occur in the food eaten in all types of household, and the nutritional consequences, while Britain adapts itself to being in the EEC. But it is also possible to project time series forward to see what a continuation of the trends of the 1960s would lead to. *All other things being equal*, this might indicate what diet would have been chosen in the near future had the United Kingdom not become a member of the EEC; these predictions can then be modified in specific cases to take account of other factors which result from membership. But this kind of prediction, useful though it can be, is fraught with potential errors: as an example, predictions from changes occurring in the late 1950s must have been that consumption of dietary staples which had been denied to us during the postwar rationing period, such as carcase meat, eggs, and sweets, would continue to rise. Although some of these changes did occur during the 1960s, the most impressive change was a switch from home-prepared to convenience foods.

Within this broad sweep, there were other quite dramatic changes. For example, within cereal products, consumption of bread, flour, oatmeal and rice declined fairly rapidly, but 'convenience' or 'luxury' cereal products such as breakfast cereals, cakes, biscuits, and puddings increased. Meat consumption increased largely because of increases in poultry and in ready-prepared meat products. The absolute amount, although not the proportion, of pigmeat (pork, bacon and ham) also increased, but other carcase meat (mutton, lamb, beef and veal) declined. The trend to convenience forms was also apparent with fish, where there was a marked increase in the amount of quick-frozen fish purchased at the expense of fresh fish. The slight increases in fruit consumption were spread through all the types identified (citrus, apples and pears, other fresh fruit, and canned fruit). The decrease in vegetable consumption was largely in potatoes; within this there was a marked trend from loose potatoes to purchases of pre-packed potatoes. There were also declines in root vegetables and pulses, and fresh green vegetables, but these were more than compensated for by increased consumption of frozen and canned vegetables. Although butter consumption increased during the decade, there was an overall decline in 'visible' fat because of a decline in purchases of margarine. Other luxury and convenience items which increased include cream and other milk products, canned soups, pickles and sauces, and instant coffee, while purchases of tea declined, as did preserves (presumably in relation to the declining purchases of bread).

Did these dietary changes bring any nutritional advantages? The overall energy intake decreased, in relation to decreasing requirements for energy. But the proportion of energy derived from fat increased steadily from 37·4% in 1956 to 42·3% in 1971, at the expense of that derived from carbohydrate. The average protein intake remained relatively constant, but within this there was a steady replacement of protein of vegetable origin by animal protein. Of the minerals evaluated for the NFS, iron declined slightly, while calcium showed little variation. Average intakes of vitamin A, riboflavin, nicotinic acid and vitamin C all increased with only thiamin and vitamin D of the recorded vitamins declining slightly.

These were the changes that the British wanted to make with their recent economic and social history. Each region of the UK was tending towards a 'London diet' or a more affluent diet (with their emphasis on carcase meats, poultry, fresh fruit and vegetables, and lower than average consumption of bread and flour, cooking fats and margarine), while retaining many of their own food preferences. The changes were, on the whole, consistent with increasing affluence, and (all other things being equal) could be predicted to have continued in the absence of EEC entry.

With this as a background, how might entry into Europe be expected to modify these changes in our diet? Perhaps the best way to consider this is to study what people already in the EEC choose, for if we are to share similar prices, availabilities and shortages of food, should we not tend to eat what they eat?

The OECD has published more or less comparable data on the total amount (i.e. in catering establishments etc. as well as households) of major foods available for consumption in most European countries since 1954. The latest available figures, which are for about 1968, have been compared to illustrate the differences between the food consumption patterns of Britain and each of the original members of the EEC. Values have also been compared with the USA, which, being one of the most affluent nations in the world, might indicate the possible diet of Europeans in the future. Similar values for 1955/56 and 1961/62, a few years before and after formation of the original Common Market have also been compared in some detail.

The broad food consumption patterns of the UK and the 'Six' have been remarkably similar, and are basically different examples of a 'western' diet. Italy has been the most exceptional with, among common foodstuffs, the highest per caput consumption of cereals, pulses, vegetables, citrus fruit and olive oil, and the lowest consumption of sugar, potatoes, total meat, offal, eggs, whole milk, butter and margarine. The USA is similar to the other five EEC countries although it consumes less cereals, potatoes and butter, and more meat (especially beef and veal, and poultry) and eggs per caput than these countries. The approximate relative position of the UK in its per caput consumption of common foodstuffs is summarised in Table 2.

TABLE 2

CONSUMPTION OF COMMON FOODS IN THE UNITED KINGDOM IN RELATION TO CONSUMPTION BY THE ORIGINAL MEMBERS OF THE EEC (1968–69)

Bread grain	Average	Beef and veal	Low
Total cereals	Average	Lamb and mutton	Highest
Sugar	Highest	Pigmeat	Low
Potatoes	High	Poultry	Average
Pulses	High	Offal	Low
Vegetables	Lowest	Total meat	Average
Citrus fruit	Lowest	Eggs	Above average
Other fruit	Lowest	Whole milk	Highest
Butter	High	Cheese	Lowest
Margarine	Low	Fish	High

Perhaps more relevant are the similar ways in which food consumption patterns changed over the last 15 years in Britain and in France, West Germany, The Netherlands, and Belgium and Luxembourg (Italy and the USA were rather exceptional), while each country maintained many of its traditional differences, as outlined below.

Cereals

Consumption of total bread cereals (wheat and rye) steadily dropped from about 250 g to 200 g/head/day. Italy however, maintained a steady intake of nearly 350 g, including pasta, while the USA maintained a steady intake of about 150 g with a comparatively large intake of other cereals such as corn (maize).

Meat

Consumption increased in all the countries mainly because of dramatic increases in poultry (although still only to half the amount eaten in the

USA) and considerable increases in pigmeat consumption. There were also slight increases in beef and offal consumption, except in the UK. Our consumption pattern has, however, remained unique in that nearly 15% is mutton and lamb (which is almost uneaten elsewhere in Europe) while our pigmeat consumption continued much lower than in all the other countries except Italy.

Fish
Consumption generally remained steady, except for increases in France and Italy which brought them to about the level eaten in the UK.

Eggs
Consumption generally rose slightly, with the UK a little above average.

Vegetables and fruit
In the UK the changes in consumption were very small. In contrast, however, there were dramatic increases in both, often by 50% or more, in nearly all the original members of the EEC. The exception has been potatoes, which showed marked declines in Belgium and Luxembourg, France and West Germany. In some cases these changes occurred during the formation period of the EEC, but more frequently the major jump was in the mid 1960s. Thus the UK (which has in this time never had a high consumption of vegetables or fruit, especially citrus fruit), now has by far the lowest consumption of all these items in any of these countries. Only for pulses did we hold an intermediate position, but these are not a major item in the diets of these countries.

Fats
Margarine consumption declined and butter consumption increased to about twice that of margarine in the UK. The consumption of these products is very variable between countries, as shown in Table 3.

TABLE 3

CONSUMPTION OF BUTTER AND MARGARINE IN SEVERAL COUNTRIES (1968)

Country	Butter (g/head/day)	Margarine (g/head/day)
Belgium/Luxembourg	27·9	40·0
UK	25·2	14·2
France	24·6	9·1
West Germany	23·0	25·5
Netherlands	8·4	53·4
USA	7·0	13·4
Italy	5·3	3·3

Milk and cheese
Consumption of whole milk in the UK remained far above the consumption in the other countries. It was however declining slightly, in common with Belgium and Luxembourg, West Germany and The Netherlands, while it increased slightly in France and Italy. Consumption of several milk products such as skimmed milk was, however, higher in several countries than in the UK. Cheese consumption rose steadily in all the countries, but was always lowest in the UK.

Nutrients
The only nutritional interpretation of these consumption data was the energy, protein and fat contents, and the proportions derived from animal and vegetable sources. These show that in 1968 the totals were very similar for each country (Table 4).

TABLE 4

NUTRIENT CONTENT OF TOTAL FOOD SUPPLIES (1968)

Country	Energy (MJ/head/ day)	Fat (g/head/day)	Protein (g/head/day)	Proportion of protein from animal sources
UK	13·3	142	88	0·61
Belgium/Luxembourg	13·2	145	89	0·56
France	13·2	147	102	0·61
West Germany	12·5	139	83	0·65
Italy	12·3	98	87	0·43
Netherlands	13·5	156	84	0·63
USA	13·4	154	95	0·72

In these 15 years, the energy content of the diet declined very slightly in the UK, while it increased in all the other countries except West Germany; this was most marked in Italy, where it rose from only 10·0 MJ/head/day in 1955/56. Fat consumption rose only slightly in the UK compared with the greater rises in all the other countries. While the total amount of protein available remained almost constant in each country, the proportion derived from animal sources increased everywhere, most markedly in Italy, France and West Germany.

This constancy parallels the great stability of food consumption differences between the various regions of Britain over the past 15 years, and the even greater stability of nutrient intakes, as shown by the National Food Survey.

Despite the lack of comparative information on very recent food consumption in Europe, some predictions are still possible. These must be that we will expect to spend a smaller proportion of our income on food, yet on average try to buy the diet now consumed by our present upper income groups. The main changes, in the UK as well as Europe, should therefore continue to be towards animal products such as meat, cheese, processed milks and, to a lesser extent, eggs. The main increases among the various meats will be in pigmeat, poultry, and meat products. There may also be a rapid rise in fruit and green vegetable consumption to bring us closer to the levels eaten in Europe, although consumption of other vegetable products, especially cereals and potatoes, will probably continue to decline. The other trend which will almost certainly continue is towards 'convenience' versions of foods such as canned, frozen, prepacked and otherwise processed foods. These include such things as meat pies, breakfast cereals, instant puddings, canned soups and sauces. It should however be noted that in 1971 when the rate of increase in food prices quickened, British housewives tended to economise mainly by buying fewer convenience foods.

These general predictions must of course be tempered to some extent by any changes which occur in the price of foods, both in relation to each other and to non-food items. They may also be affected by new regulations affecting food composition and even by metrication of package sizes and recipes. Nevertheless, it can confidently be predicted that whatever diet we choose to eat will simply provide us with different sources of the same amounts of the same nutrients as before.

ACKNOWLEDGEMENT

I am indebted to Dr D. H. Buss for his assistance with the preparation of this paper.

PART 1

NUTRITIONAL SURVEILLANCE:
AIMS AND IMPLICATIONS

CHAPTER 5

Nutritional surveillance in Britain

W. T. C. BERRY and SYLVIA J. DARKE

Department of Health and Social Security, London

INTRODUCTION

The aims of this paper are to outline the reason why the Department maintains surveillance of nutrition in Britain, to describe the nature of this surveillance and to indicate briefly the findings and the problems revealed.

REASON FOR SURVEILLANCE

A food and welfare policy which is effective in maintaining the health and wellbeing of a nation must be based on sound nutritional and economic evidence. But the results of the surveillance by which this evidence is obtained are not necessarily limited to the implementation of a *national* policy. Some problems can be dealt with more flexibly and economically by *local* health authorities. For example, in the recent Elderly Survey (Department of Health and Social Security, 1972) such malnutrition as was observed can best be dealt with locally by the provision of meals on wheels in clubs and day centres, or by domiciliary visits, but if the study had shown that the malnutrition was related to poverty, changes in national policy would be needed. Therefore one of the important objectives of surveillance is to determine the extent to which the problems revealed are more appropriate to national or to local action.

THE NATURE OF SURVEILLANCE

Hitherto much of the field work has been done by Government Departments and some by other academic departments in medical schools and universities or research groups under the aegis of the Medical Research Council. But with the implementation of the Rothschild report a new procedure will be adopted in which the Department acts as the customer and asks outside research workers to tackle the problems of surveillance. The Department will be responsible for financing the necessary studies but will be less and less involved in the field work.

Surveillance needs to be threefold in nature. First, there is a cross-sectional component, involving studies in which detailed information may be collected, on population samples that are as nearly nationally representative as is practicable. These studies provide baseline information with which the results of future studies can be compared. Second, there should be an element of continuity, either by longitudinal studies of the same individuals at regular intervals of time or by various running indices. Such indices are derived from information which is collected regularly and which is relevant either directly or indirectly to nutritional status. Third, there are special studies, to consider in greater detail either some section of the population at special risk, or the significance of some finding that is not well understood, or the prevalence of some condition not adequately revealed by other studies. Though we do not regard research as necessarily a part of surveillance, the limiting factor in much of surveillance is in fact that further research is needed before the findings can be interpreted.

Cross-sectional studies

In contrast to some countries in which all age and sex groups are investigated in a single survey, we in Britain have made separate studies of people of different ages. This has been chiefly a matter of convenience because the experts with whom we need to cooperate come from different parts of the health services. For example, in studies of the elderly we benefited greatly by collaboration with local geriatric consultants; for pregnant women we depended on the reports of the general practitioners responsible for the mothers during their pregnancy; for schoolchildren we relied on help from the school health service, and for preschool children we worked with clinic doctors of the local health authorities (Ministry of Health, 1968b). This piecemeal approach to the problems of surveillance has both advantages and disadvantages. The experts with whom we collaborate have local knowledge from which we benefit, but it is obvious that there is never in any one year knowledge of all vulnerable groups. In addition no information is obtained about the nutrition of other members of the family.

We are at the moment more or less at a standstill as far as cross-sectional studies are concerned. There are not, at present, any indications that comprehensive cross-sectional studies on a national scale would yield information importantly different from what we already have or can obtain either from running indices or from special studies.

Running indices

Various running indices are at present in use, and these (not in order of importance) are (a) the perinatal mortality rate, stillbirth and low birth-weight rates, which have the disadvantage that they depend on many factors other than nutrition, but are useful in that they can reflect changes in the situation of a 'worst-off' minority; (b) the growth rate of school-children as determined by height and weight measurements when these are made in school medical examinations; (c) the National Food Survey which records the amount of food purchased for consumption by the household for a period of one week by some 8000 families each year; (d) the Family Expenditure Survey. We also record the number of new female volunteers for blood transfusion who are rejected because their haemoglobin is below 85%. This gives some assessment (albeit very approximate) of the incidence of anaemia in women. In addition morbidity statistics, such as those obtained from the Hospital Inpatient Enquiry Study, and mortality statistics monitor the diseases of both under- and overnutrition.

Special studies

These have been made either because the interpretation of survey data is impossible until the significance of some finding has been elucidated, or because other workers report findings which are nutritionally perturbing. Since 1965 there have been investigations into the amount and kind of iron salts that could be used to restore the iron lost in milling white flour of about 70% extraction rate (Ministry of Health, 1968a); anaemia in young children (MacWilliam, 1968) and in women (Elwood 1968); the possible significance with regard to vitamin deficiencies of reported changes in the appearance of the tongue (Yudkin *et al.*, 1970; Berry and Darke, 1972); and whether there should be changes in the fortification of infant foods with vitamin D (Department of Health and Social Security, 1970). This list is not exhaustive as there have been additional studies made on a less official basis by various colleagues and other work is now in progress.

RESULTS OF SURVEILLANCE

In Britain the only age groups of the indigenous population in which some overt primary malnutrition has been shown to occur are at the two extremes of life. Among the elderly living in their own homes or with relatives, who were studied in 1967/68 (Department of Health and Social Security, 1972), rather less than 3% of the sample were diagnosed on clinical grounds as being malnourished, and in most of these individuals (over 2%) malnutrition was secondary to some non-nutritional cause. In this survey 7·6% were found to have serum alkaline phosphatase (SAP) concentrations considered to be higher than the accepted normal, and although the necessary investigations for a full diagnosis could not be made in the field, the geriatricians concluded that there was a small problem of osteomalacia especially among the housebound elderly. In addition, 57 of 778 subjects were diagnosed clinically as having angular stomatitis, but their average daily intake of riboflavin was 1·2 mg compared with 1·3 mg for those not showing the condition. The high and almost identical average intakes of the two groups suggest that much of the observed angular stomatitis was non-nutritional. It was not however possible to make a controlled feeding test with these subjects. The follow-up study of the sample of elderly people, which is at present being made, may give more information since we are able in the present study to use the appropriate enzyme reactivation test.

Among the young, and chiefly among the Asian immigrants, overt nutritional rickets has recently again been reported. After the 'scare' of hypercalcaemia in the 1950s, action was taken to reduce the level of fortification of infant foods with vitamin D and since then on average clinical rickets has been reported in about one child per 2000 from some of our industrial cities (Department of Health and Social Security, 1970). The assertion that even a small number of overt cases of what used to be known as the 'English disease', might be indicative of a more prevalent 'subclinical' deficiency of vitamin D, led to one of the special studies initiated by the Department (Stephen and Stephenson, 1971). Serum alkaline phosphatase concentrations were estimated in London children aged 2–3 years known to be receiving vitamin D supplements and in Jamaican children exposed to much more sunlight than we get here. The frequency distribution curve showed a larger than expected number of children with SAP concentrations greater than the accepted normal, and was almost identical with that of groups of children in London and in Liverpool who may or may not have been receiving supplements of vitamin D (Department of Health and Social Security, unpublished results). The children in both these cities were drawn from areas in which there are likely to be sections of the population at risk of malnutrition. Thus SAP concentrations used alone as a means of assessing the prevalence of sub-clinical vitamin D deficiency seem to be of uncertain significance. For ethical reasons, we have avoided the use of radiology as an epidemiological tool. Recent claims of 'biochemical rickets' among both Asians and the indigenous population (Cooke et al., 1973) set a problem for surveillance which the Panel on Child Nutrition already has in hand.

The results from our running indices of nutrition show that in spite of a steady improvement in perinatal and low birthweight rates, and a steady increase in growth rates of schoolchildren, there still remain environmental gradients related to social and economic circumstances and to the size of the family. While it may be tempting to ascribe these differences to nutrition, there is no certainty that this is so. Indeed, the results of our recent cross-sectional dietary studies, in so far as they have been analysed, show that the average daily intakes of energy and most nutrients including protein are not consistently less in large families or those from the lower Registrar-General (RG) classes than in the others. Only the intake of vitamin C shows a consistently steady diminution with increase in family size and fall in the scale of RG social classes. Even so, the average intake was above the recommended daily intake.

From September 1968, a previous Government cancelled the provision of a daily one third of a pint of milk free to secondary schoolchildren (aged

TABLE 1

MEAN HEIGHTS AND WEIGHTS OF SCHOOL LEAVERS IN SCOTLAND (1967–71)

| | Boys | | Girls | |
	Mean height (in)	Mean weight (lb)	Mean height (in)	Mean weight (lb)
1967	60·8	100·8	60·6	105·3
1968	60·7	99·6	60·7	104·6
1969	60·7	98·7	60·7	104·0
1970	60·7	98·5	60·8	104·2
1971	60·8	99·3	60·8	104·7

Source—Scottish Home and Health Department (personal communication).

11 years onwards) on each of the 200 or so days of the school year. Table 1 shows that there has been no significant change in mean heights and weights of the secondary schoolchildren since the cancellation of their free milk.

Yet Tables 2 and 3 illustrate that the well marked gradient of height and weight with family size and social class which existed before 1968 still

TABLE 2

MEAN HEIGHTS AND WEIGHTS OF SCHOOL LEAVERS FROM FAMILIES OF DIFFERENT SIZES IN SCOTLAND[a] 1970/71[b]

| Number in family | Boys | | Girls | |
	Mean height (in)	Mean weight (lb)	Mean height (in)	Mean weight (lb)
1	61·3	103·4	61·3	108·1
2	61·2	100·8	61·3	106·7
3	60·7	98·0	61·0	104·6
4	60·4	96·3	60·6	102·6
5	60·0	94·5	60·2	100·6
6	59·7	93·9	60·0	99·8
7 or more	59·4	92·5	59·5	97·6

[a] Excluding Aberdeen City and Aberdeen County.
   10% sample of records.
Source—Scottish Home and Health Department (personal communication).

exists. Figures for the tables were supplied to us by the Scottish Home and Health Department who analyse the information on heights and weights of their schoolchildren centrally. We in England do not.

TABLE 3

MEAN HEIGHTS AND WEIGHTS OF SCHOOL LEAVERS FROM FAMILIES OF DIFFERENT RG SOCIAL CLASS IN SCOTLAND[a] 1970/71[b]

| | Boys | | Girls | |
Social class	Mean height (in)	Mean weight (lb)	Mean height (in)	Mean weight (lb)
1	61·8	101·8	61·4	103·3
2	61·5	102·2	61·2	106·1
3	60·5	97·2	60·7	103·0
4	60·2	95·4	60·5	102·6
5	59·6	94·3	59·7	100·7

[a] Excluding Aberdeen City and Aberdeen County.

[b] 10% sample of records.

Source—Scottish Home and Health Department (personal communication).

Although the reduction in intakes of protein, calcium and riboflavin consequent upon the cancellation of secondary school milk is unlikely to have been large, it was not nil, and thus if the slower growth rate of children in large families were a reflection of their nutritional status at the time, some effect on average stature might be expected. That there has been no effect so far could be because the limiting nutrients for growth at this age are not protein, calcium or riboflavin. Other possible explanations are that some non-nutritional factor is responsible, or that an average diminution in growth rate by a minority may be masked by the majority who continue to grow faster. But the alternative and very interesting possibility has to be borne in mind, that the differences observable in relation to family size and social class at age 14 have nothing to do with nutrition or indeed any other factor existing at that age, but are the result of maximal rates of growth inexorably imposed by factors operating much earlier in life.

PRESENT PROBLEMS IN SURVEILLANCE

One of the most pressing problems stems from changes in the provision of welfare and school milk announced by the Government in October 1970. The daily half price pint of milk (or its equivalent in dried milk powder) ceased to be available to all pregnant women and children under 5 years of age from April 1971, although under the new system a larger number than before are entitled to a free pint daily. School milk was cancelled for all junior schoolchildren aged 7–11 years from September 1971 except for handicapped children and those who require milk for special medical reasons. (The interpretation of 'special medical reasons' was left flexible.)

The effects of these changes, if any, are likely to be small and to depend not only on the results of a decreased intake of the nutrients supplied by milk, but on what, if anything, is eaten instead. The Committee on Medical Aspects of Food Policy (Nutrition) appointed a panel of experts to consider how best to monitor any changes in nutritional status. Special studies have been designed, accepted by the parent Committee, financed by the Department and are being made by certain university and other research bodies. The studies include the growth of both schoolchildren and preschool children, the health of expectant mothers during pregnancy and of the babies born to them. These growth studies have been so designed that longterm surveillance can be maintained, and will also in fact serve to monitor any nutritional changes which result from our present economic and industrial problems and upon our participation in the European Economic Community.

About six weeks before the changes in welfare and school milk took place, the National Food Survey introduced questions asked of the housewife designed to estimate the quantity of fresh milk drunk at home by individual members of the household. Early results for households affected by the changes governing welfare milk indicate that in the first 12 months children under 5 years were drinking slightly more milk, and expectant mothers slightly less than before but neither change was statistically significant. For children over 5 years of age, the average milk intake remained unchanged (Table 4).

TABLE 4

MILK CONSUMPTION BEFORE AND AFTER CHANGE IN WELFARE FOODS AND SCHOOL MILK

| | Consumption of milk (pints/person/week) | |
	3 months prior to 1st April 1971	12 months after 1st April 1971
Children under 5 years	4·6	4·8
Children over 5 years	4·0	4·0
Expectant mothers	5·2	4·9
All other adult females	4·0	3·4
Adult males	3·7	3·5

Source—The figures are taken from the results of the National Food Survey (Ministry of Agriculture, Fisheries and Food, 1973).

Of other running indices, the perinatal mortality and stillbirth rates and the infant mortality rate, which have been falling for the past several decades, continued to fall during 1971.

ACTION RESULTING FROM SURVEILLANCE

If the purpose of surveillance is to provide a basis for policy in food and welfare, the criterion of success must include the extent to which decisions for action have been based upon the findings. As far as vitamin D deficiency in children is concerned, a decision not to alter the system for fortification of infant foods was based on the findings of an expert panel of the Department of Health and Social Security in 1970. The recent reports of 'biochemical rickets' and in the case of Asians of overt clinical rickets and osteomalacia to which we have already referred, may necessitate some changes in the fortification system after all. We must await the results of further special studies which have been initiated by the Department.

The nutritional deficiencies of the elderly (including vitamin D deficiency) were judged on evidence from the 1967/68 survey to be best met by local rather than by national measures and a number of recommendations were made.

With reference to iron deficiency anaemia, the work of the expert panel on Iron in Flour (Ministry of Health, 1968a) in which breads enriched with labelled iron compounds were supplied to volunteers, and to the entire families of several hundred anaemic women (Elwood, 1970; Elwood et al., 1971), has given some information about the absorption of iron from bread and of the amounts of iron needed to prevent anaemia. But whether any benefit to health would result from further fortification of foods with iron remains in doubt. We await with interest the outcome of activity in the USA in this field of enrichment.

As far as the immediate present and the future are concerned, the results of the various growth studies and other measures which we have described will be of crucial importance to national policy in relation to school and welfare milk and school meals, and to the adjustments that the nation will have to make as a result of entering the Common Market.

CONCLUSION

We feel that with the development of national surveillance the main focus of attention of nutritionists is likely to move away from the experimental animal and towards man; away from man in the laboratory and the hospital and towards man as he lives his daily life, and finally, away from parochial man and towards international man. We are sure that we have a great deal to learn from other countries, from epidemiologists and from the disciplines of sociology and economics.

REFERENCES

Berry, W. T. C. and Darke, S. J. (1972). *Age and Ageing*, **1**, 177.

Cooke, W. T., Swan, C. H. J., Asquith, P., Melikian, V. and McFeely, W. E. (1973). *Lancet*, **1**, 324.

Department of Health and Social Security (1970). *Interim Report on Vitamin D by the Panel on Child Nutrition,* Rep. pub. Hlth and med. Subj., No. 123, HMSO, London.

Department of Health and Social Security (1972). *A Nutrition Survey of the Elderly*, Rep. Hlth and soc. Subj., No. 3, HMSO, London.

Elwood, P. C. (1968). *Proc. Nutr. Soc.*, **27**, 14.

Elwood, P. (1970). *Proc. Roy. Soc. Med.*, **63**, 1230.

Elwood, P., Waters, W. G. and Sweetnam, P. (1971). *Clin. Sci.*, **40**, 31.

MacWilliam, K. (1968). *Haemoglobin Levels in Young Children*, Rep. pub. Hlth and med. Subj. No. 118, Appendix H, HMSO, London.

Ministry of Agriculture, Fisheries and Food (1973). *Household Food Consumption and Expenditure* 1970/1971, Annual Report of the National Food Survey Committee, HMSO, London.

Ministry of Health (1968a). *Iron in Flour*, Rep. pub. Hlth and med. Subj., No. 117, HMSO, London.

Ministry of Health (1968b). *A Pilot Survey of the Nutrition of Young Children in* 1963, Rep. pub. Hlth and med. Subj., No. 118, HMSO, London.

Stephen, J. M. L. and Stephenson, P. (1971). *Archs Dis. Childh.*, **46**, 185.

Yudkin, J., Norman, D. H., Wilkinson, M. E. and Berry, W. T. C. (1970). *Proc. Nutr. Soc.*, **29**, 8A.

CHAPTER 6

Nutritional surveillance in Czechoslovakia

S. HEJDA and J.MAŠEK

Research Centre of Metabolism and Nutrition
of the Institute for Clinical and Experimental Medicine, Prague

NUTRITIONAL SURVEYS

Nutritional surveys are a relatively old tradition in Czechoslovakia. Some work dates back to the period before the Second World War; this work was, however, sporadic and had no major impact. Interest in nutrition increased greatly in wartime, obviously in conjunction with rationing and because the population was threatened by nutritional deficiencies.

Systematic surveys of food consumption and the nutritional status of the population were started only after the foundation of the two Institutes of Human Nutrition in Prague and Bratislava. The Prague Institute was founded in 1951 and was headed for 20 years by Professor Mašek, before, in 1972, it became incorporated into the Institute for Clinical and Experimental Medicine the interest of which is focused on somewhat different research problems. The much smaller Slovak Institute is concerned mainly with nutritional problems pertaining to Slovakia, although the two Institutes do not have strictly defined spheres of action and they cooperate, for example, by comparing results. The Director of the Slovak Institute—Bučko—is concerned mainly with experimental dietetics. After the recent reorganisation of research, epidemiological research pertaining to nutrition and the nutritional status of the population were transferred to the Institute of Food Hygiene and Nutrition which collaborates closely and extensively with the hygiene stations in regions and districts.

In the first years after the foundation of the Institute of Human Nutrition we tried to obtain a complete and overall picture of the diet and nutritional status of the population. The majority of investigations made at that time included dietary surveys, surveys focused on clinical and biochemical measurements of the nutritional status and on some economic aspects of food consumption. Several surveys of large population groups formed the basis of the long-term plan of food consumption.

In the first half of the 1950s in our population quantitative deficiencies were occasionally still encountered. A deficient protein intake was much more frequent at that time than it is now, though even then the average consumer had an adequate energy intake. In some groups the animal protein intake amounted to only 75–100% of the recommended allowance (Hejda *et al.*, 1972). The vitamin intake, in particular of retinol (vitamin A), riboflavin and ascorbic acid (vitamin C) was frequently deficient in comparison with recommended intakes. The position was similar as regards mineral elements.

Despite these deficiencies there were relatively few signs of malnutrition and only quite exceptionally was overt malnutrition encountered. On average 12 to 20% of the healthy population had minor or subclinical signs of malnutrition. Relatively frequently we recorded pallor of the skin, follicular hyperkeratosis, hypertrophy of the lingual papillae and a very red tongue. Among subjective complaints headache and loss of appetite were most frequent. In about 1·6% of the population we recorded a low food consumption, manifest clinical symptoms of malnutrition and abnormal biochemical findings—especially a lower haemoglobin level. The serum cholesterol was low, roughly by one standard deviation, *i.e.* about 40 mg/100 ml, lower than at present.

If we compare the dietary intake in the second half of the 1950s with the present situation, we find that since that time an increase in the majority of the investigated indicators occurred, in some a considerable increase. The average energy intake in some groups of adults and in old people is excessive at present and fat consumption is far too high in the majority of population groups. It is no exception to find a fat intake which is by as much as 50% higher than the recommended allowance (Hejda *et al.*, 1972). In this connection it deserves mention that in Czechoslovakia animal fats are popular, while the consumption of oils is rising only slowly despite the intense efforts of health educationists.

In an extensive nutritional survey made in 1971 the fat intake of all population groups was higher than the recommended allowance. Fat consumption had increased more markedly than the consumption of any other nutrient. Even in some groups of children where the protein intake had not yet reached the recommended level, fat consumption was excessive. When considered in comparison with recommended intakes the food consumption of adults was greater than that of children and adolescents even in areas with a high standard of food consumption. The ascorbic acid consumption was particularly inadequate, a traditional shortcoming which has persisted for many years. The position is improving slowly but despite this at the end of winter and in spring practically all population groups have an inadequate ascorbic acid intake. Imports and sales of citrus fruit are slowly rising and in 1972 the consumption was 8 kg/head/ year, compared with 1·6 kg in 1952. The consumption of apples and locally produced fruit does not vary much and depends mainly on the harvest. Some time ago we summarised in collaboration with Ošancová (Hejda and Ošancová, 1965) work on the ascorbic acid intake of our population during the past 15 years and reached the conclusion that it was improving only very slowly. The intake was lowest in March and April when in some groups, *e.g.* old people, the serum levels were extremely low. During this period of the year it was not exceptional to record daily intakes of 10–30 mg. This was, however, not due only to socioeconomic conditions. In our experience population groups with a fairly high food expenditure had a low intake of foods which are rich sources of this vitamin merely because they did not like vegetables and fruit. Despite many years of nutrition education people often value foods differently from nutritionists. At the end of summer and in autumn ascorbic acid consumption is much higher than at other times, but even then it does not reach recommended levels in all groups. On average 40% of the ascorbic acid in the diet is provided in potatoes, 40% in vegetables and the remainder in fruit (Hejda and Ošancová, 1966). The ratio of different sources is not the same in all population groups and, for example, old people in old age pensioners' homes obtain only 5% of vitamin C from fruit. We also tried to assess ascorbic acid losses during food preparation and the net intake (Hejda *et al.*, 1965) and reached the conclusion that on average as much as 53% must be subtracted from the values given in food tables. The serum ascorbic acid was also estimated in different population groups (Hejda and Krausová, 1962; Ošancová and Hejda, 1965) and found to decline with age. In our opinion this is not a biological phenomenon but a reflection of dietary intake. Very low levels were found in old people and men engaged in heavy work. We tried to remedy the low ascorbic acid status of people who have to take their meals in communal catering facilities by enriching table salt with ascorbic acid. Although we were thus able to attain high serum levels fairly easily and at low cost, we do not consider this approach an ideal solution but rather a temporary measure; moreover table salt does not appear to be the most suitable medium for ascorbic acid.

Obesity

A serious problem in our population is obesity. Our epidemiological surveys provided evidence of a high prevalence of obesity in adult men and women. If we take 115% of the desirable weight as the criterion of obesity, at present 29% of the adult male and 47% of the adult female population are obese, while the corresponding figures 15 years ago were 10 and 42% respectively. For the evaluation of bodyweight we use our national standards (Hejda and Hátle, 1961), which are rather lenient.

The number of obese subjects is increasing steadily, as well as the mean bodyweight of our population. The high incidence of severe forms of obesity, *i.e.* above 125% of the ideal weight, and the shift of obesity to younger age groups are particularly alarming. The percentage of fat assessed by hydrostatic weighing even in subjects with a so-called normal bodyweight is higher than in the population of other countries, *e.g.* in the Scandinavian countries (Petrásek *et al.*, 1965). The prevalence of obesity is lower in Slovakia than in Bohemia and Moravia, where industrialisation is more advanced. In industrial centres there is a high percentage of obese women but not of men. This may be due to the fact that the whole family adopts the dietary habits of the head of the family who is engaged in heavy work, although in these areas a high percentage of women are not employed. The relationship between energy intake and obesity is obvious in women but not in men, probably due to different physical activity. It is interesting that the ratio of obese men and women in Bohemia and Moravia is 1:2, while it is 1:1·5 in Slovakia. The difference is probably in the type of work performed—in Slovakia more women are engaged in agricultural work and this work is less mechanised than work in industry. In women we found a high prevalence of obesity, especially in groups with a high ratio of dietary carbohydrates. A certain role in the development of obesity is played also by the frequency of food intake as we were able to prove some time ago in collaboration with Fábry (Hejda and Fábry, 1964).

We also studied psychological and sociological aspects of obesity. Many obese subjects do not know their bodyweight, or to put it more exactly, do not want to know it. Not every obese subject wants to lose weight. Some people still consider obesity a symbol of wellbeing and good health (Hejda and Ošancová, 1969). The high prevalence of obesity is, no doubt, also due to the low level of physical activity, including advancing mechanisation and automation of work.

Atherosclerosis

Another problem studied was the relationship between nutrition and atherosclerosis. In collaboration with cardiologists we investigated for several years the nutrition in two areas threatened to a different extent by ischaemic heart disease. Both areas were rural, the lowland area being more threatened than the mountainous area. In the lowland area we found higher energy intake and much higher fat consumption than in the mountainous area, although the two areas are only 60 km apart. After five years this difference increased further and in the lowland area there was a further increase in energy and fat consumption. The mean fat consumption of men as well as women was more than 140% of the recommended allowance which is about 130 g fat in men and 105 g in women. The intake of linoleic acid varies round the lower borderline of the recommended intake. The differences in fat and energy intake as well as in clinical and morphological atherosclerosis were statistically significant (Reiniš and Hejda, 1969).

Haematopoiesis

For some time we paid attention also to the relationship between nutrition and haematopoiesis. The iron intake in adults varies on average between

13 and 14 mg/day. We were unable to reveal a significant correlation between iron intake and the haemoglobin level. Significantly lower haemoglobin levels were, however, found in a group of subjects which had a concomitant lower iron and protein intake (Hejda and Ošancová, 1968).

The problem of nutritional anaemias was investigated in particular by Zamrazilová (Zamrazilová and Hejda, 1968). According to her findings in our population 8 % of the men and 10 % of the women are anaemic. The highest incidence of anaemia was recorded in women of fertile age.

We followed up, on a long-term basis, the nutrition of children in an area with fluoridated water and compared the findings with a control group. As we did not reveal any statistically significant differences we have to ascribe the 60 % reduction in the incidence of dental caries to fluoridation. At present in Czechoslovakia water is fluoridated in about 30 different large areas. In areas where water is not fluoridated children receive fluoride in tablet form. Fluoridation of food is not foreseen.

The results of a number of our investigations were used as a basis for the elaboration of recommended nutrient allowances (Hejda et al., 1972). The present allowances were adopted in 1971 and will be valid for five years. Then they will be, as agreed, revised, corrected and extended. Most probably recommended allowances of some vitamins, phosphorus and linoleic acid will be included. We also intend to introduce the factor of age and bodyweight into the recommended allowances for adults.

Despite the fact that the results of epidemiological investigations are not always applied immediately, this work is considered an important tool of preventive medicine. The results are used also in other, non-medical fields, for example in agriculture, food processing and foreign trade. They also play a part in the nutrition and price policy as well as in health education. Naturally in the national economy and in the nutrition and price policy medical and nutritional arguments are not the only ones which must be considered. As in other countries, an important part is also necessarily played by economic possibilities.

REFERENCES

Hejda, S. and Fábry, P. (1964). *Nutr. Dieta*, **6**, 216
Hejda, S. and Hátle, J. (1961). *Prakt. lékař*, **41**, 991.
Hejda, S. and Krausová, J. (1962). *Čs. gastroent. výž.*, **16**, 494.
Hejda, S. and Ošancová, K. (1965). *Die Nahrung*, **9**, 629.
Hejda, S. and Ošancová, K. (1966). *Prakt. lékař*, **46**, 182.
Hejda, S. and Ošancová, K. (1968). *Čs. gastroent. výž.*, **22**, 74.
Hejda, S. and Ošancová, K. (1969). *Čs. gastroent. výž.*, **23**, 360.
Hejda, S., Ošancová, K. and Cibochová, E. (1965). *Čs. gastroent. výž.*, **19**, 443.
Hejda, S., Ošancová, K. and Mašek, J. (1972). *Rev. Czechosl. Med.*, **18**, 101.

Ošancová, K. and Hejda, S. (1965). *Čs. gastroent. výž.*, **19**, 232.
Petrásek, R., Rath, R. and Mašek, J. (1965). *Rev. Czechosl. Med.*, **11**, 267.
Reiniš, Z. and Hejda, S. (1969). VIIIth International Congress of Nutrition Prague, Abstracts of Papers.
Zamrazilová, E. and Hejda, S. (1968). *Čas. lék. ces.*, **107**, 1496.

CHAPTER 7

Nutritional surveillance in the USA

D. M. HEGSTED

Professor of Nutrition, School of Public Health, Harvard University, Boston

I suspect that this conference will find that nutritional surveillance has never been adequate anywhere and certainly that is true of the United States. There will probably be little disagreement with the proposition that we ought to know more about nutritional status in our countries and how it is changing with time. The question we will probably not resolve, but which needs much more thought and work, is what should be done about it? Can we develop adequate systems which work but are reasonable in cost, time, and effort?

I start out this way because in the United States, at least, there has been a substantial change in attitude in the last few years. During the 1950s and 1960s the underlying attitude was that practically anything that was useful in improving the health and wellbeing of the US population was worthwhile and ultimately fundable. It seems quite clear now that this is not true—that funds available will not continue to grow—and that competition between uses for the money available will be severe. The problem, therefore, is not the relatively abstract one of whether or not we *ought* to have better data than we now have. The real questions are what will it cost, what will we actually measure, what will we do with the data once they are available, and can such programmes be sold to the funding agencies?

Even though there has never been an adequate surveillance system in the United States, it is abundantly clear that much has changed in the United States in the past 50 years. Pellagra, rickets and other nutritional deficiency diseases were serious health hazards in the 1920s and early 1930s. These became rare in the late 1930s and early 1940s. The causes of this change are not entirely known and they reflect changes in general nutritional knowledge among physicians, health officials and the general public, changes in income levels of the population, changes in the food supply, some deliberately organised nutrition programmes, and other changes. They provide, nevertheless, a dramatic example of what has been accomplished since nutrition became a subject of scientific inquiry. The problem now is more difficult in the sense that we are dealing with less dramatic problems. This is not to say that they are less important. Quite clearly, smallpox is a more important disease than the common cold, but after smallpox and similar diseases are under control the more benign diseases become increasingly important. The obvious aim is optimal health. A major difficulty is that we are concerned with many quite different conditions all of which are influenced by the kind and amount of food eaten. They range from obesity and cardiovascular disease to deficiencies of many different essential nutrients to excesses of toxic materials or potentially toxic materials. Food consumption is influenced by income, educational systems, agricultural policy, cultural background, the food industries, advertising, and many other factors. Small wonder that even the definition of nutrition surveillance is difficult.

I think it should be perfectly clear that the objective of nutritional surveillance should not be to estimate the number of individuals in a population who are suffering some disability because of an inappropriate food supply. The ultimate objective must be to anticipate and prevent developments which may lead to disability or risk of disability. This, of course, will always be a matter of judgment and thus subject to argument, disagreement, and compromise.

My approach today will be to review the major sources of information available in the United States and to comment briefly upon the findings. The major sources of information about food availability and food consumption are the US Department of Agriculture's national food consumption surveys which have been conducted at 10 year intervals for a considerable period of time, the last in 1965 (US Department of Agriculture, Reports 1–17). These include the collection of household food disappearance data and, in the last survey, individual food and nutrient intakes based upon 24-hour recall data (US Department of Agriculture, 1972). The sample studied is presumably a statistical sample representative of the US population and the last survey included some 15 000 households surveyed in four different seasons and some 15 000 individual dietary histories. These kinds of data are supplemented, of course, by a variety of studies on small selected groups which have been reported in the literature. Many of these have been summarised by Davis et al. (1969) and by Kelsay (1969).

Summaries of the Ten State Nutrition Survey have now appeared (Center for Disease Control, 1972). This survey represents the first attempted national evaluation of nutritional status. Ten states were selected and in these some 24 000 families were randomly identified from census enumeration districts of the 1960 census in which the average income was in the lowest quartile. Since the sample was drawn randomly from these enumeration districts, not all of the families were poor. The sample is not representative of the United States population but can be assumed to be about as representative of the low income groups in these states as can be achieved. Approximately half of the 86 000 individuals in the families identified participated in the examination. This included a medical history, physical examination, anthropometric measurements, X-rays of the wrist, haemoglobin and haematocrit, and dietary information. Selected subsamples of infants, young children, adolescents, pregnant and lactating women and people over 60 years of age received more detailed biochemical and dietary evaluation. Unwillingness to have blood drawn or otherwise participate limited the sample size in some of these groups.

A survey of approximately 3500 preschool children presumed to represent a cross-sectional sample of the population which included biochemical examination as well as dietary data has been partially reported (Owen *et al.*, 1969; Owen *et al.*, 1971). These kinds of general surveys are supplemented, of course, by many smaller studies reported in the literature. These have been summarised by Davis *et al.* (1969) and Kelsay (1969).

Finally, I should mention that a National Health and Nutrition Survey is now in progress. This is patterned after the Ten State Survey and is expected to include approximately 15 000 individuals per year from a randomly selected sample of the United States population. No official reports are yet available.

TEN STATE SURVEY

I wish first to present briefly the findings of the Ten State Survey since these are the only comprehensive data available and then discuss these conclusions relative to other reports.

Physical findings

Clinical examinations are relatively unproductive in United States surveys. Signs and symptoms of most mild nutritional deficiencies are non-specific and clear-cut nutritional deficiencies are rare and unlikely to be observed in randomly selected samples. No adequate system for reporting hospital experience exists but it is certain that classical deficiency diseases are infrequently found. It should be noted, however, that a few cases of permanent disability such as may be caused by Wernicke's syndrome and Korsakoff psychosis in alcoholics impose a tremendous burden, financial and otherwise. Better systems of recording the experience of hospitals and practising physicians are needed.

The physical and anthropometric data do expose some interesting findings—some expected, some not. As expected, obesity is a substantial problem. From 5 to 25% of adult men and from 10 to 55% of adult women were classified as obese. Obesity was more prevalent in black women and less prevalent in black men than in whites. Higher income was associated with more obesity in men but not necessarily in women. The prevalence of obesity in adolescents ranged from 5 to 33% and was not clearly related to income. Obesity in both adults and children appears to be inversely related to social class and income (Goldblatt *et al.*, 1965; Moore *et al.*, 1962; Stunkard *et al.*, 1972).

An unexpected finding was that although the median heights and weights in children were not too far from those expected from the Stuart–Meredith standards there was a substantial excess of small children. Thus, from 18 to 46 % of the children surveyed fell below the 15th percentile for height and a similar number below the 15th percentile for weight. The excess of small-for-age children was greater at younger ages. The number of such children was larger in poor families but not limited to low income families. Although black families were generally poorer, black children tended to be taller and more advanced in skeletal age than white children.

It is not clear what these findings mean. Since the trend in the United States has been for the population to get taller and larger and since the standards were established some years ago, one might have expected the opposite finding. There is the possibility that some of the findings may simply reflect the grouping of the children into age groups. If the groups cover too wide an age range, the younger children will appear to be too small and the older children too large. Also, it is known that there is a substantial excess of infants with small birthweights in the poverty groups and the heights and weights of young children will reflect these to some degree. A number of questions are raised. Are the conventional standards now in use satisfactory? How does one deal with infants with small birthweights in cross-sectional surveys? Are special standards needed for the evaluation of the black population?

Another major problem underscored by the survey was the prevalence of dental caries, periodontal disease and poor oral hygiene. Although this may be considered to be only partially a nutritional problem, it is related to the nature of the food eaten and the adequacy of the fluoride intake. Many communities do not have a fluoridated water supply although it is clear that this will cut the caries rate in half. Many communities have essentially no dental care. Many communities simply cannot provide appropriate treatment because of the costs and lack of trained people.

Biochemical findings

The interpretation of biochemical findings is and will continue to be controversial. The methods are not as accurate or consistent as they should be and standards are not as well defined as they ought to be. However, I would emphasise again that the objective is not to identify the number of individuals who are malnourished. Rather, the objective should be to identify individuals or populations at risk. Obviously, preventive programmes cannot be maintained if we assume that nutrition programmes are only required when significant evidence of clinical deficiency can be found. At the same time, the standards must not be set unrealistically high so that time, effort, and money are wasted in programmes which yield no benefit. Informed judgment is the only method of arriving at appropriate standards.

The biochemical methods and the standards of evaluation were essentially those used by the Interdepartmental Committee on Nutrition for National Defense (1963). The inadequacies of many of these are rather well known but, unfortunately, not much has been done in the last decade to develop better methods or improved standards. It is also regrettable that nutrition surveys have, more or less, become locked into a pattern of looking at a few traditional nutrients and the scope of nutrition surveys remains limited. Although I cannot review the evidence today, I wish to mention the evidence that such nutrients as zinc, magnesium (Flink and Jones, 1969), chromium, pyridoxine (Luhby et al., 1971; Sauberlich et al., 1972) and vitamin E (Davis, 1972) may be of public health significance (Mertz and Cornatzer, 1971). We are bogged down in traditional methodology and may well be overlooking problems which are more important than some of those we study.

The most surprising biochemical finding was the large number of individuals with low levels of plasma vitamin A (retinol). Considering 20 μg/100 ml as 'low' (some risk of vitamin A deficiency) and 10 μg/100 ml as 'deficient' (high risk of vitamin A deficiency), nearly 50% of the children in the American–Mexican population of the southwest were below the 20 μg level. Intakes were also low since this is largely a 'corn and bean' population. Up to 10% of the age-sex groups identified had levels below 10 μg. Fewer but significant numbers of low plasma values were observed in many other areas. Children generally had lower levels than adults.

Xerophthalmia is apparently not known in this population but lesser degrees of physical disability and changes in dark adaptation, for example, do not appear to have been adequately studied. Plasma levels in this southwest population are not too different from those found in Central America where clinical disease is readily recognised.

The second major problem identified was iron deficiency anaemia. According to the standards used (Table 1) the problem is widespread in all ages and sexes and all parts of the country although it is more prevalent in poor groups and in blacks and Spanish-Americans compared to whites. It should be emphasised that the standards used were considerably more severe than those recommended by the World Health Organization (1972) yet up to 8% of some groups were classified as 'deficient'. Although serum iron values were not consistently obtained, it is apparent that most such individuals had low levels. It is surprising that a relatively large proportion of adult men were classified as 'deficient'.

Although the arguments and counterarguments about standards and the programmes needed are recognised, we conclude that iron deficiency is a problem of real public health significance in the United States.

As might be expected very low vitamin C (ascorbic acid) levels in the plasma (<0.1 mg/100 ml) were found in 2 to 5% of individuals in various age–sex groups and up to 10 to 20% had levels below 0.2 mg/100 ml. Urinary riboflavin levels judged to be low or deficient were found in similar numbers. Both of these measures are known to be relatively 'labile' and do not necessarily identify individuals who are at risk over any period of time.

TABLE 1

HAEMOGLOBIN DEFICIENT AND LOW VALUE
CLASSIFICATIONS (g/100 ml)

Age and sex	Deficient	Low
<2 All	<9.0	$9.0-9.9$
2–5 All	<10.0	$10.0-10.9$
6–12 All	<10.0	$10.0-11.4$
13–16 Male	<12.0	$12.0-12.9$
13–16 Female	<10.0	$10.0-11.4$
>16 Male	<12.0	$12.0-13.9$
>16 Female	<10.0	$10.0-11.9$

Plasma albumin levels were somewhat surprising. Very few individuals were classified as 'deficient' according to the standards used (Table 2), yet relatively large numbers—up to 20% in some age–sex groups—had levels somewhat below normal. Low income groups had larger numbers with reduced levels than high income groups.

TABLE 2

SERUM ALBUMIN DEFICIENT AND LOW VALUE CLASSIFI-
CATION (g/100 ml)

Age	Deficient	Low
<1	Standard not available	<2.50
1–5	Standard not available	<3.00
6–16	Standard not available	<3.50
>16	<2.80	$2.80-3.49$

Low levels of thiamin excretion were rarely found. Although goitre was observed, it did not appear to be related to low iodine consumption as judged by iodine excretion levels.

TABLE 3

RELATIONSHIP BETWEEN BIOCHEMICAL TEST AND INTAKE IN 12–14-YEAR-OLD CHILDREN[a]

Quartile according to biochemical test	Iron (mg) Male	Iron (mg) Female	Intake Protein (g)	Vitamin A (iu)	Vitamin C (mg)	Riboflavin (mg)	Thiamin (mg)
1	<12·4	<12·0	85	3 756	52	1·6	1·4
2	12·7	12·3	90	4 401	55	2·0	1·3
3	13·6	13·1	87	4 937	75	2·1	1·4
4	>14·0	>13·4	85	4 663	98	2·4	1·4

[a] Compiled from data in Ten State Survey.

Food and nutrient consumption

Nutrient intake might be considered to be the most sensitive measure of nutritional inadequacy since there is little doubt that inadequate intake → tissue depletion → biochemical lesion → clinical deficiency. Yet, estimations of nutrient intake cannot identify the individuals at risk of nutritional deficiency. I believe that this is because dietary histories cannot be taken accurately enough to reflect the *usual* intake of individuals, however they are done. In addition, there is little doubt that individuals react differently to similar diets.

It is also my conviction that dietary histories give reasonable estimates of the intake of *groups* of people and this is true whether one uses relatively inaccurate 24 hour recall data or more sophisticated and presumably more accurate measures. One can legitimately compare Group A with Group B however these are defined or compare time trends in a population. It is easy to show that, for example, the Mexican-Americans in the United States have lower vitamin A intakes than a neighbouring population. However, on an individual basis the correlation between intake and biochemical findings is either nil or disappointingly low.

The data in Table 3 were obtained by dividing the populations into quartiles according to the biochemical finding and then calculating the average intakes of the four groups. Presumably thiamin and protein show no correlation because protein is rarely limiting in the diets and because the error in the thiamin excretion data is large compared to the range of intakes. The correlation with vitamin C is relatively high because the range of intakes is large and the plasma level is responsive to immediate past intakes. The correlation with vitamin A is poor because the errors in estimating vitamin A intake are large and the serum level more nearly represents usual intakes than current intakes. It is of interest that in both boys and girls there was an apparent correlation in haemoglobin level and iron intake.

It is worth emphasising, I think, that the accuracy of dietary histories varies greatly depending upon the nutrient under study. The intake of vitamin A, for example, may vary from practically nil on one day to 10 000 to 20 000 iu on another depending upon whether green and leafy or yellow vegetables were eaten. Also, the vitamin A content of those high carotene foods varies greatly from sample to sample. On the other hand, protein intakes and iron intakes tend to be considerably more constant and are fairly closely related to energy intake.

US DEPARTMENT OF AGRICULTURE NUTRIENT AND FOOD CONSUMPTION SURVEYS

I cannot begin to summarise these extensive publications and will content myself with a few remarks about them. These data are invaluable for

US DEPARTMENT OF AGRICULTURE, WASHINGTON, D.C.

Nutrients less than the recommended dietary allowances[a]

Sex	Age (years)	Protein (%)	Calcium (%)	Iron (%)	Vitamin A value (%)	Thiamin (%)	Riboflavin (%)	Ascorbic acid (%)
Male and female	Under 1			30 or more				
	1–2			30 or more				
	3–5			11–20				
	6–8							
Male	9–11		1–10					
	12–14		11–20	21–29				
	15–17		1–10	1–10		1–10		
	18–19							
	20–34		1–10					
	35–54		11–20					
	55–64		11–20					
	65–74		21–29					
	75 and over				1–10		11–20	1–10
Female	9–11		21–29	30 or more		1–10		
	12–14		21–29	30 or more	1–10	1–10		
	15–17		30 or more	30 or more		11–20		
	18–19		21–29	30 or more		1–10		
	20–34		21–29	30 or more	1–10	1–10	1–10	
	35–54		30 or more	30 or more		1–10	11–20	
	55–64		30 or more			1–10	1–10	
	65–74		30 or more	1–10	1–10	11–20	11–20	
	75 and over		30 or more	1–10	11–20	11–20	21–29	

[a] NAS-NRC, 1968, US diets of men, women and children, 1 day in Spring, 1965.

many purposes. They show trends in consumption of foods and nutrients, and changing dietary patterns, and how these relate to such variables as income group, cost of foods and area of the country. These are important in terms of general policy and help to explain or predict current and future developments.

The major problem that I have already touched upon is how they can or should be used in nutritional surveillance. Table 4 is taken from the publication on individual nutrient consumption and shows the number of individuals whose intakes (24 hour recall) were below various standards. I am convinced that this is not really an appropriate way to treat the data even though this is exactly what we would like to know. As I have already mentioned, the accuracy of the data as a measure of usual intake varies greatly depending upon the nutrient under study. If intake varies greatly from day-to-day or week-to-week, an excess of 'low' diets will inevitably be found. Data on vitamin A intake are inevitably poorer than those on nutrients whose intake is more uniform. Iron and protein contents of diets are relatively uniform and are about 6 mg Fe/1000 kcal (4184 kJ) and 40 g protein/1000 kcal (4184 kJ) in the United States. Errors in estimating the consumption of these kinds of nutrients are more likely to be in the amount of food consumed than the kind. In any event, the number of individuals who are represented as being below standard may be more a reflection of the errors in the methodology than anything else. I have suggested an approach which might make such data more useful in nutritional surveillance at least for some nutrients (Hegsted, 1972).

OTHER REPORTS

As already indicated summaries of literature reports dealing with dietary intakes and biochemical findings have been prepared by Davis *et al.* (1969) and Kelsay (1969). Although these vary substantially in their conclusions, the groups studied were markedly different, the techniques utilised differed, and the objectives were often quite different. One can conclude that the general impression obtained from such isolated reports supports the conclusions of the Ten State Survey.

I want to comment specifically on a couple of problems. Repeated reports suggest that folate deficiency may be a substantial problem in the United States, particularly in pregnant women (National Research Council, Food and Nutrition Board, 1970). However, there is substantial disagreement on the interpretation of biochemical findings. This is a high priority area that needs serious consideration. Questions regarding zinc, pyridoxine and some other nutrients that I have already mentioned fall into a similar class but have attracted less clinical interest.

It is my firm conviction that the major nutritional problem in the United States is coronary heart disease. At least two-thirds of American men and a less well-defined proportion of women have circulating levels of cholesterol and other lipids that are undesirably high. This has long been recognised as a major risk factor and can be modified by dietary manipulation. The best evidence indicates that modification of the dietary fat would be the most acceptable way to lower blood lipids. Although we do not deny that many factors are no doubt involved in this problem, it is unfortunate that arguments among the so-called 'experts' serve to prevent action programmes. Modification of the mortality and morbidity rate from coronary disease should be a major health objective in the United States and most countries, and the problem is so serious that we cannot wait for the ultimate resolution of all of the questions that need answering. The upper class in many of the developing countries are rapidly developing patterns of food intake that can be predicted to result in similar epidemics of heart disease.

At least one other problem should be of major concern to nutritionists in the United States. This is the unsatisfactory outcome of pregnancy among the less privileged groups. While this is no doubt a complex problem involving poor or inappropriate medical care and the nutritional correlates are not well defined, it is a major problem. Means of evaluating nutritional status during pregnancy are poorly developed.

NUTRITIONAL SURVEILLANCE

The development of adequate surveillance systems present formidable challenges. The collection of data in itself is of little value unless it leads to identification of specific problems and solutions. Broad surveillance systems may fail to do this.

For example, in the Ten State Survey some 32 000 blood samples were examined for haemoglobin. This must be considered to be a respectable number. It represents about 0·016% of the population of the United States, and since the sample was drawn from the lower income quartile, it should represent about 0·064% of that population. However, the data are not very meaningful unless they are examined in terms of specific age groups and with regard to sex, ethnic groups, income, region of the country, etc. Other groupings may, of course, be even more meaningful. However, the point I wish to make is that by the time the data were divided into the various groups, the numbers often became too small for an accurate evaluation of differences.

We must be careful that we do not get caught up in a numbers game. A 1% incidence in the population may be a very important problem and, if concentrated in a particular area or age–sex group, might represent a rather large proportion of that group. Large, randomly arranged surveys may well fail to identify where the problem is and will be unlikely to obtain enough information to relate it to causal factors or suggest appropriate solutions. Many of the nutrition problems must be assumed to be regional and often concentrated in minority groups. If so, solutions are likely to be local rather than national. The time required for conducting and evaluating large surveys is often so long that they are outdated before they are published and are primarily of historical interest.

I believe that although national data are helpful and may be especially important in a political sense, the best solutions will eventually be found in the incorporation of appropriate methods in local or regional institutions (White House Conference on Food, Nutrition and Health, 1970). Such systems should also utilise a great deal of information that is routinely collected or could be routinely collected in operating health centres of various kinds. Finally, a system must be developed in which there is a feedback of information to those who can and should utilise it on a day-to-day basis. Nutritional surveillance systems must be developed to improve the nutritional status of our population and not to fill tomes in the archives.

REFERENCES

Center for Disease Control (1972). *Ten State Nutrition Survey* 1968–70, DHEW Publ. No. (HSM) 72–8134, Atlanta, Georgia.

Davis, K. C. (1972). *Am. J. clin. Nutr.*, **25**, 933.

Davis, T. R. A., Gershoff, S. N. and Gamble, D. F. (1969). *J. Nutr. Ed.*, **1**, 41.

Flink, E. B. and Jones, J. E. (1969). *Ann. N.Y. Acad. Sci.*, **162**, 705.

Goldblatt, P. B., Moore, M. E. and Stunkard, A. J. (1965). *J. Am. med. Ass.*, **192**, 1039.

Hegsted, D. M. (1972). *Ecology of Food and Nutrition*, **1**, 255.

Interdepartmental Committee on Nutrition for National Defense (1963). *Manual for Nutrition Surveys*, 2nd ed., US Government Printing Office, Washington, D.C.

Kelsay, J. L. (1969). *J. Nutr.*, **99**, Suppl. 1, Part 2, 123.

Luhby, A. L., Brin, M., Gordon, M., Davis, P., Murphy, M. and Spiegel, H. (1971). *Am. J. clin. Nutr.*, **24**, 684.

Mertz, W. and Cornatzer, W. E., editors (1971). *Newer Trace Elements in Nutrition*, Marcel Dekker, New York.

Moore, M. E., Stunkard, A. J. and Strole, L. (1962). *J. Am. med. Ass.*, **181**, 962.

National Research Council, Food and Nutrition Board (1970). *Maternal Nutrition and the Course of Pregnancy*, National Academy of Sciences, Washington, D.C.

Owen, G. M., Garry, P. J. and Kram, K. M. (1969). *Am. J. clin. Nutr.*, **22**, 1444.

Owen, G. M., Garry, P. J., Lubin, A. H. and Kram, K. M. (1971). *J. Pediat.*, **78**, 1042.

Sauberlich, H. E., Canham, J. E., Baker, E. M., Raica, N. and Herman, Y. F. (1972). *Am. J. Clin. Nutr.,* **25,** 629.

Stunkard, A. J., d'Aquili, E., Fox, S. and Filion, R. D. L. (1972). *J. Am. med. Ass.,* **221,** 579.

US Department of Agriculture. *Household Food Consumption Survey* 1965–66, Report Nos. 1–17, Agriculture Research Service, Washington, D.C.

US Department of Agriculture (1972). *Food and Nutrient Intake of Individuals in the United States, Spring* 1965. *Household Food Consumption Survey* 1965–66, Report No. 11, Agriculture Research Service, Washington, D.C.

White House Conference on Food, Nutrition and Health (1970). *Final Report,* US Government Printing Office, Washington, D.C.

World Health Organization (1972). *Nutritional Anaemias,* WHO Technical Report Series No. 503, Geneva, Switzerland.

APPENDIX

Excerpted from Hegsted, D. M. (1972). *Ecology of Food and Nutrition,* **1,** 255.

The differences in observed nutrient intakes must come from three sources: real differences in the *usual* intake, the day-to-day variations in intake and the errors in the dietary history. If the latter two are essentially random errors, some progress can be made in defining *usual* intakes, at least with some nutrients.† As has been shown in Fig. 5, the data upon protein intakes show a reasonably *normal* distribution and the standard deviation falls as the period of investigation is prolonged. The total variance in the observed protein intakes (T^2) can be

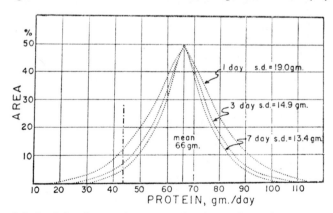

Fig. 5. Calculated distribution of protein intakes from 1-*day,* 3-*day and* 7-*day dietary records.*

† The author wishes to thank Dr Jacob J. Feldman, Department of Biostatistics, Harvard School of Public Health, for suggestions and discussion on the treatment of dietary data.

assumed to consist of the differences in the *usual intakes* of the individuals examined (σ^2) and an error term (s^2) representing day-to-day variations and the simple errors in the dietary history. Thus, for the 1-day data

$$T^2 = \sigma^2 + s^2$$

or

$$19^2 = \sigma^2 + s^2$$

and for the 3-day data

$$14 \cdot 9^2 = \sigma^2 + s^2$$

Solving the two simultaneous equations

$$361 = \sigma^2 + s^2$$
$$180 = \sigma^2 + s^2$$
$$\sigma^2 = 152 \quad \text{and} \quad \sigma = 12 \cdot 3$$

Similarly, if one solves for differences between the 1-day and 7-day records, $\sigma = 12 \cdot 2$, approximately the same value.

Thus, Fig. 5 has been modified as shown in Fig. 6 to include distribution of usual intakes. It may not appear that a standard deviation of 12·2 is appreciably different from that of the 7-day histories which is 13·4 g/day. However, we must remember that we are primarily concerned with the tail-end of the distribution curves. The distribution of *usual intakes* indicates that only 2% of the diets were below the RDA which does have a different connotation than 4%. If the approach used by Beaton were applied to these data on *usual intakes*, the prevalence of deficiency would fall to negligible proportions.

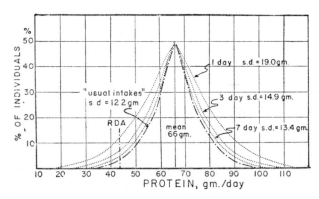

Fig. 6. Figure 5 modified to include the distribution of 'usual intakes' (see text for discussion).

CHAPTER 8

Nutritional surveillance in Canada

J. A. CAMPBELL

*Acting Director, Nutrition Bureau, Department of National
Health and Welfare, Ottawa*

The need for information on the nutritional status and dietary intake of
Canadians has been recognised for some time. While surveys have been
conducted on specific groups of the population, the Canadian Council
on Nutrition, as early as 1964, recognised the need for a comprehensive
national survey. Finally, in 1968, plans were laid by the then Food and Drug
Directorate of the Department of National Health and Welfare for a
nationwide survey to be carried out. Field operations began in September
1970 and ended in October 1972. It is the purpose of this paper to review
the basis for the survey and outline plans for nutritional surveillance and
nutrition programmes in Canada.

NEED FOR THE SURVEY

Up to 1968 there had been several reports indicating that certain segments
of the Canadian population might not be as well fed as has been assumed
(Campbell, 1970). These reports related primarily to eating patterns of
schoolchildren and senior citizens.

Evidence obtained by our Research Laboratories (Hoppner *et al.*,
1968; Hoppner *et al.*, 1969) indicated that approximately 10% of human
liver samples collected at necropsy in an Ottawa hospital contained no
vitamin A. In Vancouver the figure was 2% and in Montreal it was 22%.
The absence of hepatic stores of the vitamin was strongly suggestive of
inadequate intake or utilisation of vitamin A. It was further reported
(Canadian Council on Nutrition, 1968) that 400 cases of rickets were
admitted in 1967 and 1968 to three hospitals in Montreal and Toronto.
The cost of hospitalisation in one hospital alone in Quebec was estimated
at a third of a million dollars per year.

These reports suggested a need for more detailed information about our
nutritional status. In addition we also had to take cognisance of our changing food habits and their possible impact on our nutrient intake. In the
past, our food intake was largely, if not entirely, composed of traditional
foods with their original nutrient content. Now, as a result of the decrease

in activity in practically all segments of the population, there is a resultant decrease in intake of foods such as cereals and potatoes. The demand for prepackaged, precooked and other types of convenience foods seems to be increasing. There is a trend away from three normal meals a day consisting of the traditional food groups. There is also an increasing interest in the development of substitutes for traditional foods such as milk and meats. Finally, there is increasing and significant use of new formulated foods including snack foods and so-called 'instant' meals, particularly by certain groups of the population. We were thus faced with several factors which might significantly modify our nutrient intake and thus the nutritional adequacy of our diet.

We were also concerned about the intake of additives and contaminants by the Canadian population. We had no information on the consumption of foods by individuals or by various segments of the population. The survey was therefore planned with the objective of providing basic information on the nutritional wellbeing of Canadians for the planning of public health programmes and for the development of Food and Drug Regulations. To accomplish this, it was proposed to:

1. estimate the prevalence of nutritional diseases and disorders in groups of the Canadian population characterised by geographical location, type of community, income level and the age–sex and physiological state of the individuals;
2. identify the types and quantities of food ingested by individuals in these groups to determine the level of ingestion of nutrients, food additives, non-nutritive substances and pesticide residues.

FEASIBILITY STUDY

Since this was the first attempt at a national nutrition survey in Canada and because of the logistic and administrative problems involved, a feasibility study was undertaken in 1969. In the course of this study, the participation of the provincial departments of health was secured and the interest of universities and other organisations in nutrition was assessed. Groups of experts were assembled to advise on specific subjects including, survey design and sampling, methodology for assessing the dietary intake, the clinical picture and the biochemical nutritional status, and standards to be used in data interpretation. It was planned that provincial departments of health would play a major role and maximum use would be sought of all university and other personnel interested in nutrition. The local public health units would have a particularly important place in obtaining the cooperation of individuals in the community and in follow-up on persons found suffering from malnutrition.

PLAN FOR THE SURVEY

The main survey was based on the following design characteristics:

1. The survey covered the civilian, non-institutional population of the ten provinces.
2. Data were to be available on five regions, Atlantic, Quebec, Ontario, Prairies and British Columbia.
3. Three types of area varying in population density were identified, metropolitan, urban and rural.
4. Two income levels were identified, *i.e.* above and below an income of $2500 for a family of two with $500 increments for each additional person.
5. The first level of sampling involved enumeration areas which were selected to give an estimate of seasonal variation by obtaining two matched samples. Enumeration areas (EAs) contain 400 to 1600 individuals, depending on population density.
6. The second level of sampling was households which were selected from lists of all households for each enumeration area.
7. Individuals to be examined were drawn at random for ten age–sex categories, based on limits of 5, 10, 20, 40 and 65 years.
8. Eighty EAs were allocated to each region, 40 in each of two season surveys. Thus, there were 400 for the whole of Canada. With 50 persons per day being examined in each EA, the total sample for this part of the survey was 20 000. In addition, 1000 pregnant women were examined.

The selection procedure permitted the calculation of the probability of selection of each person in the sample and allowed for the calculation of survey estimates and estimates of sampling variability.

The personnel of each survey team operating survey centres numbered about 24 and comprised advance party interviewers, medical examiners, anthropometrists, dental examiners, dietary interviewers, and necessary support staff.

In addition to the main survey, plans were also made to sample about 2500 Indians living on reservations and 800 native and white people in the Yukon and Northwest Territories. The sampling of Indian reservations took into account the presence of six cultural groups in the five socio-economic regions used by Nutrition Canada and the fact that some reservations are near population centres and some are remote from such centres. For isolated areas, the team was reduced to eight to facilitate travel and accommodation. A special survey was also designed to examine 500 transient youth in several metropolitan areas.

DATA OBTAINED

Each subject selected or entering the survey was given a clinical assessment, along with anthropometric and dental examinations, and blood and urine samples were taken. With the exception of haemoglobin and haematocrit measurement on blood, and sugar and albumin on urine, which were made in the field at the time of examination, all biochemical measurements were carried out in the central laboratories in Ottawa. Nineteen separate determinations were performed on the blood and urine samples using automated systems. The dietary questionnaire detailed the food eaten the day before the examination. In addition, a food frequency form was filled out which listed a large number of foods such as soft drinks, milk, formula meals, cereals, beer, and sought to find the number of servings per day, week or month. This information is to be used for estimating the food additive or food contaminant load which some people may reach.

Data have been tabulated on a regional and provincial basis. They are being reviewed by an Advisory Committee on Data Interpretation, on which both departmental and other scientists are represented. The committee is also charged with putting forward recommendations for appropriate action.

It is planned that data on each province will be discussed with the province involved on a confidential basis and then released when data on all provinces are complete later this year. This will be followed by a national report in 1974.

Considerable thought and discussion was given to various ways of expressing the data. We were fully cognisant of the problems to be encountered under designations such as 'deficient' and 'normal'. On the other hand, it was recognised that some judgment must be made of the data, otherwise the Data Interpretation Committee was not fulfilling its duty. It was finally decided to list the proportion of the sample for the various strata under three categories, low risk, medium risk and high risk. These categories, which would apply to clinical and biochemical data, would include those individuals for whom there is a low, moderate, or high probability that malnutrition exists or is developing. Dietary data are being presented in cumulative frequency charts.

USE OF DATA

Now, having completed the survey, the question arises—how will the results be used? Obviously we will have a record of the proportion of the population at risk as judged by the various criteria. If a significant proportion of the population were found to be at risk in terms of vitamin A status, there may be some justification for increasing the vitamin A content of certain widely used foods. Any necessary action could be taken by amending present food standards in the Food and Drug Regulations.

Other types of data may indicate that certain groups of the population are not consuming available nutritious foods. The answer may lie in promoting information on these foods or in developing improved nutrition education methods aimed at specific groups *e.g.* the primary school group. If deficiencies are found in significant numbers in any group, region, income level or population density level, there would obviously be a need for more detailed investigative work. Such would be included in our nutritional surveillance programme which I will discuss briefly.

The present survey should also serve as a baseline for an evaluation of any enrichment or other intervention or education programmes which may be considered necessary. Data on food intake by persons in the ten age–sex categories will indicate the types of food they are consuming. At a given time they will show trends with age as to the use of various types of foods such as new snack foods, substitute foods and traditional foods. The data on nutrient intake may suggest whether or not problems are likely to be encountered.

Data on food consumption and particularly on food frequency will permit definition of the levels which foods contribute not only nutrients, but also food additives and contaminants. Use has already been made of data on fish consumption to determine the possible intake of mercury from this source by the Canadian population and the possible risk that this may be to their health.

NUTRITIONAL SURVEILLANCE

With the completion of Nutrition Canada we will have an estimate of the nutritional status and dietary intake of Canadians as of 1972–73. The question then arises, where do we go from here? We have already taken steps to ensure that maximum use will be made of Nutrition Canada data. Funds are being set aside for the use of researchers and provincial departments who may wish to seek more information from the data bank.

We have also discussed with the provinces a proposal for continued surveillance on a cooperative basis with them. The objectives of this proposal are threefold:

1. follow-up evaluation of specific nutritional disorders in segments of the population found to be malnourished by Nutrition Canada;
2. evaluation of public health and nutrition education programmes to ensure their effectiveness in the protection of the nutritional health of Canadians;

3. monitoring of the nutritional health of the people of Canada to detect changes in eating patterns and to assess the consequences of such changes on health.

To meet the stated objectives, a surveillance system is being designed to assess the various aspects of nutrition. These include medical and dental examinations, biochemical determinations and anthropometric measurements as well as evaluation of dietary patterns of Canadians.

To ensure the acceptability of the programme among Canadians and to enlist their participation, it was felt that the surveillance system should combine a service function along with survey techniques. Obviously the efficient combination of these techniques will require considerable developmental work and the close coordination of the surveillance system with the health care delivery system at the community level.

Finally, in order to provide a focus for nutrition activities at the federal level, a Nutrition Bureau was set up last year. The Bureau has three main functions, nutrition surveillance, nutrition programmes and nutrition evaluation. The surveillance group will coordinate field activities which includes liaison with provincial departments of health and through them with local health units or community health centres. This group will be responsible for the training of personnel involved in surveillance work, for conducting biochemical analysis and for data processing.

At the provincial level there should exist close liaison between the nutrition surveillance group and the local health services in the provincial department of health. This liaison should ensure the participation of the local health units or community centres. This participation will be in the form of commitment of staff to surveillance activities.

In addition to surveillance, the Nutrition Bureau will act as a coordinating centre for nutrition information and education programmes. In this work, it will assist provinces and local health units in the testing and evaluation of nutrition education methods and will coordinate and integrate the work of public health nutritionists across Canada.

The Bureau will also be responsible for a variety of projects including: a revision of the Canadian Dietary Standard; the compilation of the nutrient content of Canadian foods; the assessment of food production and consumption data, and nutritional labelling policy.

SUMMARY

Data from Nutrition Canada should permit an accurate assessment of nutritional status and dietary intake of all segments of the Canadian population at this time.

The surveillance programme planned in cooperation with provincial and local health groups should assure the continuing assessment of the nutritional health of Canadians and of the nutrient content of the food supply.

The formation of the Nutrition Bureau will furnish a means of coordinating nutrition programmes and activities at both federal and provincial levels in Canada.

ACKNOWLEDGEMENT

The author is deeply indebted to Dr Z. I. Sabry who carried out the Feasibility Study for the survey, acted as National Coordinator for Nutrition Canada and developed plans for surveillance programmes.

REFERENCES

Campbell, J. A. (1970). *Can. J. Pub. Health*, **61,** 156.

Canadian Council on Nutrition (1968). *Canadian Nutr. Notes*, **24,** 85.

Hoppner, K., Phillips, W. E. J., Murray, T. K. and Campbell, J. S. (1968). *Can. med. Ass. J.*, **23,** 983.

Hoppner, K., Phillips, W. E. J., Erdody, P., Murray, T. K. and Perrin, D. E. (1969). *Can. med. Ass. J.*, **101,** 84.

PART 2

INFANT FEEDING:

HOW SPECIALISED A PRODUCT IS NEEDED?

CHAPTER 9

Breast feeding

MAVIS GUNTHER

Esher, Surrey

For the period, presumably of many millions of years, during which the young of our forbears have been fed entirely on their mothers' milk in the first part of their lives, the processes of survival of the fittest must have been at work. Human milk has presumably evolved along with human beings and we can take as a basic assumption that the milk's composition has been well tried. The questions now arise: what qualities and components of the milk are specifically suited to the baby's needs; which should be borrowed in designing substitute milk feeds and can the recipe be improved?

Human milk is complete enough as a food for a baby to double or even treble his birthweight without additions. It must therefore contain the whole gamut of essential foods that nutritionists know about, and probably others not yet recognised. It does not necessarily follow that it can be totally relied on as a recipe of the perfect food for all babies. If one keeps to the evolutionary argument, there is no reason to suppose that the milk has been tested and evolved to suit the needs of premature babies. Without modern feeding aids almost all would have died at the outset. It has been an empirical finding that very few babies weighing under 2·5 kg at birth can feed well enough from the breast for survival. Now that even very small babies live to become normal healthy adults, there is a need for a more specialised product or for additions to be made to human milk to meet the circumstances.

The amount of protein in milk decreases continually from the high value, sometimes even 10%, at parturition to about 2% a week later and it continues to fall very slowly to approximately 1% or less at a year. Human milk of similar composition has been obtained from mothers in peacetime USA and wartime Britain, from starving mothers in concentration camps and from Indian mothers with low protein intake. The amount of protein increases at the end of a lactation, when the scanty last secretion, regression milk, comes to resemble colostrum, and it also goes up briefly if the mother develops acute intramammary mastitis. Analyses of other components in the milk should be accepted with caution if the protein content of a sample is out of step with the usual estimate for that stage of lactation. Analysts have to be aware that those who obtain or give samples of milk may be doing so because the baby is not being put to the breast for a reason in itself associated with altered composition. There appears to be little clinical justification for matching the protein content of bottle feeds to that of late milk but, if breast feeding is taken as a pattern, the present day recommendation of stronger and stronger feeds as the baby grows is out of step.

In composition, human milk protein contains relatively and absolutely less casein than cows' milk but approximately similar amounts of the milk serum proteins. On electrophoresis human casein separates into three components which can be subdivided into several more immunologically. The three fractions have different amino acid compositions and other chemical qualities.

While the chemist thinks of the structure and differentiation of the protein components, the paediatrician concerns himself more with some of their specific effects or freedom from them. The immunological qualities of the milk are, to my mind, far more important than any others to human babies. They come under three headings: the antibodies in the colostrum and milk, the augmentation of their activity by iron-binding proteins and lysozyme, and the milk's freedom from antigenic activity within the species.

In 1892 Ehrlich demonstrated that antibodies in mouse milk were absorbed unaltered into the circulation of the suckling mouse (Ehrlich, 1892). When the almost quantitative absorption of colostrum globulin by calves in the first 48 hours was recognised, some doctors hurried to assume that colostrum had the same importance in humans. And when the newborn baby was found to have received antibodies across the placenta while *in utero* and to have no easily measured increase in circulating antibodies after taking colostrum, opinion swung: colostrum was said to have no value except as a purgative. It should be said in parentheses that it is not a purgative and there seems to be no basis for wishing a baby to receive one. The interest in colostrum in calves diverted attention from the fact that human *milk* contains antibodies, in titres lower than those in colostrum and of the same specificities as those in the mother's serum.

The first clear evidence that the antibodies were effective as antibodies against infection, and were not merely a chance offering of edible protein, came in the study of oral immunisation against poliomyelitis. In this form of immunisation a living attenuated non-paralytic form of the virus is fed to the baby. For lasting protection of the baby there must be a 'take', an active infection which results for a while in living virus being present in the stools. This fact provided a reliable means of measuring whether or not immunity was being produced. Kenny *et al.* (1967) found that where the baby was breast fed and the mother's serum carried antibodies to poliomyelitis, the baby was not infected by the oral dose. Although this uncertainty of immunisation can be vexing to the would-be immuniser, the difficulty can be overcome simply enough by giving the baby an extra dose of vaccine when lactation ends. But the significance of the work is that antibodies in breast secretion are, without doubt, effective in giving some protection to a baby against viral infections, provided that the mother has antibodies to that virus. The large surveys by Douglas (1950) and by Mellander et al. (1959) showed lower incidences of measles and rubella among breast-fed babies. The sites of infection by the different viruses and the sites of protection may not be certain. The antibodies, mostly as IgA in the colostrum and milk, have been found in the faeces and presumably can be active throughout the length of the gut. They would also join, or perhaps stand in for, the IgA secretion of the naso-pharynx. There is little doubt that although the experimental evidence relates to poliomyelitis virus, the antibodies of milk reduce infection by others.

The recognition of the importance of antibacterial antibodies has a different history. Glynn (1969) showed that *Escherichia coli* antibodies plus lysozyme and complement could lyse *E. coli in vitro*. This seemed to begin to explain the lower risk of gastroenteritis in breast-fed babies but it is the partnership of the antibodies with lactoferrin (the second form of protective protein) which is now believed to be the principal controlling mechanism of growth of bacteria in the gut (Bullen et al., 1972). Lacto-ferrin, an iron-binding protein related to transferrin, constitutes between a tenth and a third of the protein in breast secretion. Bullen et al. (1972) have shown that its power to bind iron denies iron to bacteria, inhibiting their multiplication. This power is greatly enhanced by the presence of antibodies to the bacteria concerned and can be annulled by the addition of iron. These important recent discoveries bring secondary considerations. These proteins are active in the intestine and some lactoferrin is to be found in the stool: it must be escaping digestion. Antitrypsin, a protein, is also present in colostrum and milk and is likely to be protecting against digestion. All three classes of protein, the antibodies, lactoferrin and antitrypsin, are denatured by heat. Cooked or uncooked, they serve as food and there is an attractive neatness about the dual use in the ordinary course of events.

Turning now to milk proteins as antigens: it would be wise to assume that there are genetic differences in the structure of the proteins of human milk. If so, their possible antigenicity must be low. Sera from 100 infants tested against two samples of milk contained no detectable antibodies to any constituent. This is in contrast to cows' milk proteins given by mouth. In a study, 71 out of 92 babies given two or more bottle feeds in the first three months were found to have made antibodies to the proteins. The strength of the antibodies to the component proteins varied from baby to baby (Gunther et al., 1962). Several practical aspects relating to the anti-genicity of cows' milk proteins need to be considered. In the same investi-gation, the milks given to the babies, whatever the brand, had been heat treated and were still highly antigenic: denaturation offers no escape and there seems to be no advantage in altering the proportions of the proteins. There is the hypothesis that some cot deaths are due to anaphylactic shock in sensitised babies who have aspirated milk into their lungs. Whether many or no cot deaths are brought about by this mechanism, the fact remains that whey proteins—not casein—have been specifically detected in the lung parenchyma after cot death (Parish *et al.*, 1964). For the time being, until the part allergy may play in cot death is clearer, an increase in the proportion of whey proteins in a feed seems undesirable. On the other hand, casein given in too high a concentration has been known to form in the stomach and intestine solid masses which need surgical treatment. The possibility has been considered of adding high titre swine anti-*E. coli* antibody or bovine lactoferrin to infants' feeds. Each may have a use but each may be antigenic.

Both the quantity and the composition of the fat in human milk are of concern to those designing milks for infants. Estimation of the amount of fat obtained by a baby in a day presents special difficulties. Fore-milk contains less fat than hind-milk; the proportion of hind-milk depends on the degree of emptying; the milk ejection reflex is not always sustained in proportion to the fullness of the breast. Where the breast has been emptied to a more or less standardised end point at zero hour and at each milking, the proportion of fat is found to vary diurnally (Gunther and Stanier, 1949). Only estimates taken from 24 hour samples starting from a zero hour emptying are useful. My preference is to take 2·8 % for early milk and 3·8 % for mature milk (Macy and Kelly, 1961).

The fatty acid composition of human milk fat has some consistencies in its variation. Acids of shorter length than C_{10} are hardly present (0·26 %) whatever the stage of lactation or the mother's diet (Insull and Ahrens, 1959). Lauric ($C_{12:0}$) and myristic ($C_{14:0}$) acids are present in the fat of secretion before delivery, increase in amount in the first postpartum days and are present even if the mother eats virtually no fat, being synthesised in the gland. Palmitic ($C_{16:0}$) and perhaps palmitoleic ($C_{16:1}$) are thought to be derived from diet and synthesis (Read and Sarrif, 1965). The amounts of the acids beyond C_{16} by contrast are affected by the diet, taking days rather than hours to reach a full effect. In a detailed study of one mother on known intakes (Insull *et al.*, 1959), the oleic acid constituted 42·6 % and linoleic and linolenic together 10·3 % after a week of eating 123 g lard daily, changing to 28·7 % oleic and 42 % linoleic and linolenic after three weeks of a high intake of corn oil. Some 17 acids of C_{20} or more make up 5 % of the total in the milk of mothers on diets of their own choice.

Undoubtedly the milk of mothers consistently taking different diets must result in different fat compositions in their babies. The question remains whether or not the variation perhaps in some parts of the body— the brain, bone marrow or adrenal for instance—alters the baby's life prospects. The composition of human milk and other infant foods are not alone in their responsibility: Hansen *et al.* (1970) found the fatty acid composition of foetal brains from Uganda and Denmark to be different. The maternal diet had had an effect before birth.

The lactose, mineral and water content of milk need to be considered together. Mammary gland secretion and blood are isotonic and are the same in humans and cows. Although the baby's kidney can deal with rather more than isotonic solutions the concept of isotonicity serves as a landmark. The osmolar load is made up principally by the lactose, sodium and potassium. The metabolism of the lactose results effectually in a hypotonic drink. Adding sugar to slightly diluted cows' milk presents the baby with less spare water when the sugar has been metabolised and with an initial hypertonic solution in the stomach.

One must suspect that when a baby is given a milk with high protein (and consequent high urea) and high sodium he will experience thirst and drink more. He would then gain more weight and the clinician is left to decide whether the greater weight means that the bottle-fed baby was growing too fast or that the breast-fed baby was receiving too little. Levin *et al.* (1959) found that if the sodium in human milk was made equal to that in a cows' milk mixture by the addition of salt, babies gained weight faster, and not only in the initial stage when sodium retention was suspected.

As far as we know, traces of every item of the mother's diet are secreted in human milk—including unchanged protein molecules. Kon and Mawson (1950) and many others have charted the range of variation of several vitamins, providing a basis for standards in other milks. I would like to point out that it appears from Kon and Mawson's record of the ascorbic acid amounts in one woman's lactation that the mother depletes her reserves unless her intake is about 50 mg a day. At this intake, which may be taken as physiological, the baby was receiving something like 40 mg divided between all feeds (which might be regarded as a saturation level). As ascorbic acid participates in corticosteroid secretion we should probably take the hint from breast milk and keep near to a saturation level in babies.

Infection is antagonistic to good nutrition and nutritionists should be willing to think whether scantiness or intermittency of folic acid and of its central portion *p*-aminobenzoic acid can protect just as sulphonamides and septrin can sometimes cure some infections. Hawking (1954) has shown that *p*-aminobenzoic acid is needed by the malaria parasite for its multiplication. In his work a monkey feeding her baby was given a diet containing none while her baby was inoculated with the parasite and no multiplication of the parasites occurred. A single dose of *p*-aminobenzoic acid to the mother was followed by a brief multiplication of the parasites in the baby and then their failure. It seems that in malarious areas the random eating by the mothers of food containing *p*-aminobenzoic acid would result in a central population of surviving babies who had developed active immunity in this way from multiple abortive infections. The extremes would have died from lack of immunity or too great an infection. If absence can prevent malaria it is similarly likely to inhibit bacterial infections such as streptococcal ones. Preparation of milk for infant feeding should not permit excessive bacterial formation of folic or *p*-aminobenzoic acids even though sterilisation is going to kill the bacteria.

I have called my contribution 'breast feeding' rather than 'human milk' because the processes of feeding as well as the composition need to be considered. If, again, you will allow as evolutionists that feeding has evolved to be mostly successful, then one should look with respect at the constraints imposed by behavioural limits involved. Babies have innate rules about what they will accept. In a totally primitive society without benefit of grinding or sieving a baby would be protected from taking anything but breast milk until the age of seven or eight months. Normally a baby does not accept lumps of food until that age. This happens to be when the baby is beginning to be steady when sitting up and may have some teeth; it seems a reasonable timing of the coming of a natural skill. Of course you can teach a baby to swallow lumps earlier—and recognise the items on the nappy afterwards—or dodge the refusal by making food smooth; then you can give him starch. A baby would not normally be given water and I have seen very young hungry babies spit it out with anger. We do not know how far thirst and hunger are differentiated in babyhood; recipes should not involve a baby's recognition of the need for more water.

The limitation of the baby's intake to human milk, which would have been the primitive baby's lot over some months, had the great advantage of defending him from notions. The loving mother, the distraught mother, the scientist and the manufacturer all cast round for something extra to give him—to make him sleep or to make the food more like an adult's choice. Providing the mother is well fed and the secretion ample there seems to be little scope for improvement apart from the addition of vitamin D to human milk; even that would probably not be necessary where light can irradiate the fatty secretions of the areola.

The protective qualities of human milk are peculiar to it and they will not be artificially reproducible in the near future. Fairly simple modifications of cows' milk are known to nourish a baby well. We need many investigations of long term effects of modifications before we can be confident about them. The exceptional needs of premature babies call for special modifications of human or cows' milk.

REFERENCES

Bullen, J. J., Rogers, H. J. and Leigh, I. (1972). *Br. med. J.*, **1**, 69.
Douglas, J. W. B. (1950). *J. Obstet. Gynaec. Br. Empire*, **57**, 335.

Ehrlich, P. (1892). *Z. Hyg. Infect Krankh.*, **12**, 183.

Glynn, A. A. (1969). *Immunology*, **16**, 463.

Gunther, M. and Stanier, J. E. (1949). *Lancet*, **2**, 235.

Gunther, M., Cheek, E., Matthews, R. H. and Coombs, R. R. A. (1962). *Int. Archs Allergy appl. Immun.*, **21**, 257.

Hansen, I. B., Clausen, J., Somers, K. and Patel, A. K. (1970). *Acta neurol. scand.*, **46**, 301.

Hawking, F. (1954). *Br. med. J.*, **1**, 425.

Insull, W. and Ahrens, E. H. (1959). *Biochem. J.*, **72**, 27.

Insull, W., Hirsch, J., James, T. and Ahrens, E. H. (1959). *J. clin. Invest.*, **38**, 443.

Kenny, J. F., Boesman, M. I. and Michaels, I. H. (1967). *Pediatrics, Springfield*, **39**, 202.

Kon, S. K. and Mawson, E. H. (1950). *Human Milk*, Spec. Rep. Ser., med. Res. Coun. Lond., No. 269. HMSO, London.

Levin, B., Mackay, M. M., Neill, C. A., Oberholzer, V. G. and Whitehead, T. P. (1959). *Weight Gains, Serum Protein Levels, and Health of Breast Fed and Artificially Fed Infants*, Spec. Rep. Ser., med. Res. Coun. Lond., No. 296. HMSO, London.

Macy, I. G. and Kelly, H. J. (1961). In *Milk: the mammary gland and its secretion*, **2**, p. 265. Edited by S. K. Kon and A. T. Cowie, Academic Press, New York.

Mellander, O., Vahlquist, V. and Mellbin, T. (1959). *Acta paediat., Stockh.*, **48**, suppl. 116.

Parish, W. E., Richards, C. B., France, N. E. and Coombs, R. R. A. (1964). *Int. Archs Allergy appl. Immun.*, **24**, 215.

Read, W. W. C. and Sarrif, A. (1965). *Am. J. clin. Nutr.*, **17**, 177.

CHAPTER 10

Artificial feeding, especially in relation to composition of infant foods in Britain and the EEC

ELSIE M. WIDDOWSON

Dunn Nutritional Laboratory, Cambridge

The weeks or months just after birth are the only time of life when we live on a single food. This is also the time of life when faulty nutrition may be expected to have its greatest effect. It is of prime importance, therefore, that the food given to the young baby is as perfect as science and technology can make it. Breast milk has been described as the only natural food, and before the mid-eighteenth century in Britain, if a mother could not breast feed her baby and a wet nurse was not available, the baby died. This may still be the position in many developing countries today. In the developed countries, however, there are now hundreds of preparations on sale as dried powders or liquids that vie with each other as being the best possible food for babies. Some of them are essentially whole, or partially defatted, cows' milk. Some have lactose or other carbohydrates added. Some use whey, a by-product of the cheese industry, as the base, and in some all the fat originally in the milk may be removed and replaced with a mixture of other fats.

I thought it might be helpful to find out what babies in European countries other than our own were being offered as their daily fare. The description on the tins or packets was not very informative, so we decided to analyse the preparations ourselves. We have analysed one tin or packet each of 30 dried milk preparations from seven European countries. We have been told that these are among the leading brands. Table 1 gives a list of these foods, the names of the manufacturers and the country of origin. The parent company of some manufacturers is in a country other than the one where the food is made and sold. Pelargon and Eledon, both Nestlé products, are made and sold under the same trade name in more than one country. They may or may not have the same composition. Three milks, Farilacid, Prodieton and Swiss Eledon are acidified preparations. Some foods are numbered 1 and 2. This indicates that No. 1 is designed for the young baby, No. 2 for the older one.

TABLE 1

MILKS ANALYSED

Country of origin	Code no.	Name of milk	Manufacturer
UK	GB 1 and 2	Ostermilk 1 and 2	Glaxo
UK	GB 3 and 4	Cow & Gate 1 and 2	Cow & Gate
UK (USA)	GB 5	SMA	John Wyeth
France	F 1 and 2	Lait Guigoz 1 and 2	Guigoz
France	F 3	Nativa	Guigoz
France	F 4	Galliasec 1	Gallia
France (UK)	F 5 and 6	Milumel 1 and 2	Milupa (Glaxo)
France (UK)	F 7 and 8	Lemiel 1 and 2	Milupa (Glaxo)
Holland	NL 1	Almiron B	Nutricia
Holland	NL 2	Farilacid	Nutricia
Holland	NL 3	Frisolac	Co-op Condens-fabriek Friesland
Holland (USA)	NL 4	Similac	M & R Laboratories (Ross Labs.)
Germany	D 1	Milumil	Milupa
Germany	D 2	Nan	Nestlé
Italy (Switzerland)	I 1	Pelargon	Nestlé
Italy (Switzerland)	I 2	Prodieton	Nestlé
Italy	I 3	Plasmolac	Plasmon
Italy	I 4	Auxolac	Carlo Erba
Denmark (Switzerland)	DK 1	Eledon	Nestlé
Denmark (Switzerland)	DK 2	Pelargon	Nestlé
Switzerland	CH 1	Eledon	Nestlé
Switzerland	CH 2	Pelargon	Nestlé
Switzerland (France)	CH 3	Guigolac	Guigoz
Switzerland	CH 4 and 5	Humana 1 and 2	Galactina & Swiss Milk Co.

CARBOHYDRATE

Breast milk has a higher percentage of lactose than cows' milk, and the first stage in the 'humanising' of cows' milk was to increase the carbohydrate in it, either by adding more lactose or by including other carbohydrates. Table 2 shows the percentage of carbohydrate in the milk powders in our series that contained only lactose. As far as we could tell only three, Ostermilk 2, Cow & Gate 2, and Swiss Eledon have no added carbohydrate at all. Ten have lactose added and among them are the other

TABLE 2

CARBOHYDRATE IN MILKS CONTAINING LACTOSE ONLY
(g/100 g powder as monosaccharides)

	Name	Code no.	Lactose
No carbohydrate added	Ostermilk 2	GB 2	39
	Cow & Gate 2	GB 4	37
	Eledon	CH 1	48
Lactose added	Ostermilk 1	GB 1	64
	Cow & Gate 1	GB 3	63
	SMA	GB 5	55
	Nativa	F 3	54
	Frisolac	NL 3	57
	Similac	NL 4	54
	Nan	D 2	64
	Plasmolac	I 3	51
	Humana 1	CH 4	54
	Humana 2	CH 5	56

TABLE 3

CARBOHYDRATE IN MILKS CONTAINING CARBOHYDRATES OTHER THAN LACTOSE
(g/100 g powder as monosaccharides)

Name	Code no.	Lactose	Sucrose	Glucose	Fructose	Maltose Dextrins Starch	Total
Lait Guigoz 1	F 1	25	38	—	—	—	63
Lait Guigoz 2	F 2	22	34	—	—	—	56
Galliasec 1	F 4	28	30	—	—	—	58
Almiron B	NL 1	8	30	—	—	22	60
Milumil	D 1	23	28	—	—	13[a]	64
Pelargon	I 1	29	14	—	—	17[a]	60
Prodieton	I 2	23	23	—	—	20	66
Auxolac	I 4	28	14	—	—	19	61
Eledon	DK 1	28	27	—	—	10	65
Pelargon	DK 2	31	15	—	—	15[a]	61
Pelargon	CH 2	30	16	—	—	13[a]	69
Guigolac	CH 3	38	—	—	—	24	62
Farilacid	NL 2	23	—	25	—	15[a]	63
Milumel 1	F 5	32	15	6	3	5[a]	61
Milumel 2	F 6	37	11	6	3	5[a]	62
Lemiel 1	F 7	28	12	9	4	8[a]	61
Lemiel 2	F 8	39	11	5	2	5[a]	62

[a] Starch reaction with iodine in KI.

three milks on sale in Britain. Table 3 shows what carbohydrates have been added to the other 17 milks. Sucrose and dextrimaltose are the most common additives, but four French milks include invert sugar from honey. It is clear from Tables 2 and 3 that the Eledons on sale in Denmark and Switzerland are not the same. Nine of the 12 milks containing 'dextrimaltose' or 'predigested starch' gave a positive starch reaction with iodine in potassium iodide.

One of the Dutch products Almiron B, which holds a large part of the market in Holland, contains only 8% lactose, and the sucrose and dextrimaltose amount to more than 50% of its weight. Carbohydrate provides more than half the energy in 14 of the milks. In human milk carbohydrate provides about 40%.

PROTEIN

Total protein in the milk powders ranged from 10 to 29%. The percentage varies inversely with the amount of carbohydrate that has been added, and depends also on the manipulation of the fat.

Four of the milks, Nativa from France, Almiron B and Frisolac from Holland and Nan from Germany, are based largely on whey with small amounts of skimmed milk, and they have a lower proportion of casein and a higher one of whey proteins than cows' milk. In Nativa and Almiron B the percentage of the protein contributed by casein is about 40 and therefore similar to that in human milk. In Frisolac and Nan only 10–20% of the protein is contributed by casein. All other milks have the cows' milk pattern of proteins in which casein makes up 85% of the total.

FAT

A fundamental change that is sometimes made when cows' milk is 'humanised' is to remove the milk fat and replace it with other fats or oils. This goes back to 1919 when Gerstenberger and Ruh (1919) published a paper in the United States describing a preparation which they called Scientific Milk Adaptation, SMA, in which they substituted a mixture of cod liver oil and beef tallow for the milk fat. The milk fat was no doubt made into butter and sold as a by-product. The fat mixture was chosen so that its iodine number was the same as that of breast milk fat. This preparation evidently survived until 1935, for Dr Emmett Holt tested it then, and showed that the fat in it was very poorly absorbed by babies (Holt et al., 1935); this was because it contained more of the less readily absorbed long

chain saturated fatty acids than does breast milk fat and less of the unsaturated ones. The name 'SMA' has stuck, but the fat mixture has changed,
and the SMA now on sale in Britain consists of skimmed milk with added
lactose, vitamins and iron, and a mixture of animal and vegetable fats
chosen to make the fatty acid composition similar to that of breast milk
(Widdowson, 1965).

Sixteen of the present series of milks have had the cows' milk fat partly
or entirely replaced with other fats. The object is twofold. The first is to
improve the absorption, for cows' milk fat has been known for many years
to be poorly absorbed by young babies (Holt *et al.*, 1935) and a failure
to absorb fat may lead to a poor absorption of calcium (Southgate *et al.*,
1969). This failure to absorb calcium, often associated with a high intake
and absorption of the phosphates in cows' milk, has been reported to lead
to hypocalcaemia and tetany (Oppé and Redstone, 1968; Widdowson,
1969; Barltrop and Oppé, 1970). The second object in replacing all or part
of the cows' milk fat with oil is to increase the polyunsaturated fatty acids,
particularly linoleic acid which is present in much smaller proportions in
cows' milk than in human milk.

TABLE 4

FAT IN MILKS CONTAINING ONLY COWS' MILK FAT

Name	Code no.	Fat (g/100 g)
Ostermilk 1	GB 1	19·2
Ostermilk 2	GB 2	26·6
Cow & Gate 1	GB 3	14·3
Cow & Gate 2	GB 4	24·2
Lait Guigoz 1	F 1	10·3
Lait Guigoz 2	F 2	17·3
Galliasec 1	F 4	10·0
Milumel 1	F 5	13·5
Milumel 2	F 6	15·5
Lemiel 1	F 7	14·8
Lemiel 2	F 8	17·3
Prodieton	I 2	9·0
Auxolac[a]	I 4	18·0
Eledon	CH 1	14·4

[a] Supplemented with linoleic acid.

Table 4 shows the percentage of fat in the 14 milks that contained only
cows' milk fat; one of these, Auxolac, had supplementary linoleic acid.
Table 5 shows the range for the 16 milks that contained plant or animal
fat. The values varied from 9 to 31 % and the percentage of energy derived
from fat from 20 to 50.

TABLE 5

FAT IN MILKS CONTAINING PLANT OR ANIMAL FAT

Name	Code no.	Fat (g/100 g)
SMA	GB 5	27·4
Nativa	F 3	28·1
Almiron B	NL 1	20·5
Farilacid	NL 2	8·5
Frisolac	NL 3	23·5
Similac	NL 4	22·7
Milumil	D 1	12·0
Nan	D 2	24·6
Pelargon	I 1	14·2
Plasmolac	I 3	20·4
Eledon	DK 1	9·1
Pelargon	DK 2	13·5
Pelargon	CH 2	11·8
Guigolac	CH 3	13·5
Humana 1	CH 4	25·6
Humana 2	CH 5	31·0

TABLE 6

SATURATED FATTY ACIDS IN MILKS
(g/100 g total fat)

Name	Code no.	C_{10}	C_{12}	C_{14}	C_{16}	C_{18}
SMA	GB 5	1	10	6	16	11
Nativa	F 3	2	9	9	22	7
Almiron B	NL 1	0	0	<1	11	2
Farilacid	NL 2	2	2	9	25	14
Frisolac	NL 3	<1	6	3	32	4
Similac	NL 4	2	19	7	9	3
Milumil	D 1	1	4	7	35	8
Nan	D 2	2	4	11	31	9
Pelargon	I 1	2	2	8	24	11
	DK 2					
	CH 2					
Plasmolac	I 3	2	2	8	25	8
Auxolac	I 4	2	2	8	26	10
Eledon	DK 1	2	3	8	27	9
Guigolac	CH 3	1	6	3	33	6
Humana 1 and 2	CH 4 and 5	1	7	4	23	8
Cows' milk fat		3	2	11	26	13
Human milk fat		2	6	9	23	8

Table 6 shows the distribution of the saturated fatty acids in milks with plant or animal fat or additional linoleic acid, with values for cows' milk and human milk fat at the bottom. Almiron B had no measurable amounts of C_{10}, C_{12} or C_{14} and less C_{16} and C_{18} than most of the others. The two milks of American origin, SMA, and particularly Similac, have a high proportion of $C_{12:0}$, lauric acid. This suggests that they contain coconut oil, and in fact they are known to do so. Similac, like Almiron B, was notable for its low percentage of palmitic and stearic acids, but all except one product had less stearic acid than cows' milk.

TABLE 7

UNSATURATED FATTY ACIDS IN MILKS
(g/100 g total fat)

Name	Code no.	$C_{16:1}$	$C_{18:1}$	$C_{18:2}$	$C_{18:3}$
SMA	GB 5	1	29	24	2
Nativa	F 3	1	35	13	1
Almiron B	NL 1	<1	27	58	2
Farilacid	NL 2	2	35	7	1
Frisolac	NL 3	0	38	16	0
Similac	NL 4	0	19	40	<1
Milumil	D 1	1	32	10	0
Nan	D 2	2	24	16	1
Pelargon	I 1	1	30	16	1
	DK 2				
	CH 2				
Plasmolac	I 3	2	47	6	<1
Auxolac	I 4	1	37	11	<1
Eledon	DK 1	1	25	22	2
Guigolac	CH 3	<1	38	14	<1
Humana 1 and 2	CH 4 and 5	<1	44	13	<1
Cows' milk fat		3	32	2	<1
Human milk fat		3	36	8	<1

Table 7 gives the values for the unsaturated fatty acids. All except two have considerably more of their fat as linoleic acid ($C_{18:2}$) than either human or cows' milk, and Almiron B and Similac are again particularly striking in this connection. From its fatty acid composition the fat in Almiron B appears to be maize oil and nothing else. The manufacturers of this milk are clearly making no attempt to mimic the fatty acid composition of human milk fat, but are using a fat found by experience to be well absorbed by young babies, even premature ones, and in which linoleic acid comprises more than half the total.

INORGANIC CONSTITUENTS

The milks were analysed for sodium, potassium, calcium, magnesium, phosphorus, iron, copper and zinc. Since the amount of milk taken by a baby is determined largely by its energy value, the amounts of the inorganic constituents have been calculated on an energy rather than a weight basis, and this enables comparisons to be made with human milk. It is generally agreed that a full term baby requires about 120 kcal (500 kJ)/kg bodyweight/day during the period after birth when it is likely to be living only on milk.

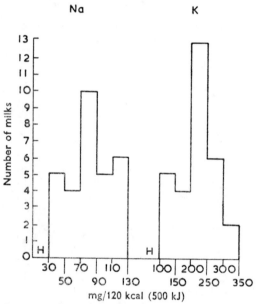

Fig. 1. *Frequency distribution of Na and K in milks (H = human milk).*

Figure 1 shows the frequency distribution of the amounts of sodium and potassium/120 kcal (500 kJ) in the milks, and therefore the approximate intakes of these electrolytes from the milks/kg bodyweight/day. Human milk provides about 25 mg Na and 90 mg K on the same basis. The values for the dried milks are all higher than this. Six milks have more than 110 mg Na/120 kcal (500 kJ). These are the two full cream milk powders, Ostermilk 2 and Cow & Gate 2, the two French preparations Milumel 1 and 2, the Swiss version of Eledon, which is made from buttermilk, and Italian Auxolac. The milks that use whey as the major source of protein would have had far more sodium and potassium than this had the whey not been demineralised by electrodialysis or some other means. Taitz and

Byers (1972) and Shaw *et al.* (1973) have emphasised the danger to young babies if they are given more sodium in their food than their kidneys can excrete with the volume of water available, and this can happen because mothers tend to use too much milk powder rather than too little when they are making up feeds (Taitz and Byers, 1972).

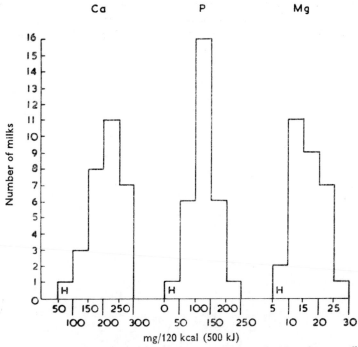

Fig. 2. Frequency distribution of Ca, P and Mg in milks (H = human milk).

Two milks contain more than 300 mg K/120 kcal (500 kJ). Potassium is excreted more readily by the infant's kidneys than sodium, and there is no reason to suppose that the amounts in these milks cannot be removed in the urine.

Figure 2 shows the frequency distribution of calcium, phosphorus and magnesium in the milk powders. All contain more calcium/120 kcal (500 kJ) than human milk, which has 55 mg. The milks that are based on whey have the least calcium. The milk containing the most calcium, Swiss Eledon, with 300 mg/120 kcal (500 kJ), also has the most phosphorus and magnesium, as well as the most protein. It is unlikely that the large amounts of calcium in some of the milks will confer any disadvantage. Whether they confer any advantage depends on the amount and kind of fat, and on the amount of phosphorus. The ratio of calcium to phosphorus, which is 2·2 in human milk, varied from 1·2 in the cows' milk preparations to 2·7 in French Nativa and Dutch Almiron B and Farilacid.

Only Almiron B contains as little magnesium as human milk (6 mg/120 kcal). Swiss Eledon contains the most (27 mg/120 kcal).

Sixteen of the 30 milks have not had iron added. These included all five from Switzerland, seven of the eight from France, three of the four from Holland and one of the two from Germany. Figure 3 shows that these milks have between 0·04 and 0·2 mg Fe/120 kcal (500 kJ). Human milk has 0·08 mg.

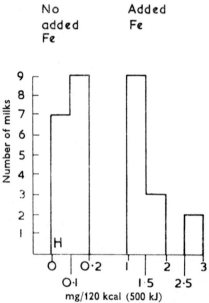

Fig. 3. *Frequency distribution of Fe in milks with and without added Fe (H = human milk).*

All five milks on sale in Britain have added iron. Iron is also included in all the milks from Denmark and Italy, and in Nativa from France, Farilacid from Holland and Nan from Germany. The fortified milks contained between 1·2 and 2·9 mg/120 kcal (500 kJ), and would provide these amounts daily per kg of bodyweight. The total amount of iron in the body of a baby weighing 3·5 kg at term is about 320 mg. If the concentration of iron in the body is to be maintained while the birthweight is being doubled the baby needs to absorb over 2 mg a day or 0·4 mg/kg. An intake of 0·2 mg or less/ kg bodyweight will clearly not enable it to do so. All the preparations containing added iron would provide the baby with more than 0·4 mg/kg a day in its food; on the milks containing the least the baby would be able to maintain the concentration in its body if it absorbed one-third of its intake. Whether it is better to add iron to infant formulae, or leave it to the mother to give to the baby separately is an open question. It is possible that additional iron in the milk may do more harm than good by saturating all the lactoferrin in the dried milk so that this is no longer effective against *E. coli* (Bullen *et al.*, 1972).

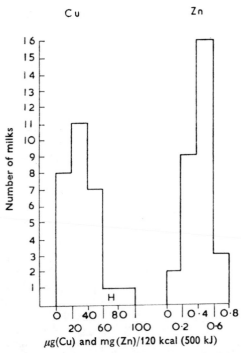

Fig. 4.   Frequency distribution of Cu and Zn in milks (H = human milk).

Figure 4 shows the frequency distribution of copper and zinc per 120 kcal (500 kJ). Cows' milk contains less copper than human milk. SMA and Nativa appear to have added copper, and possibly also Frisolac. This brings the value into the same range as the amount per 120 kcal (500 kJ) in human milk (70 μg). The liver at birth contains considerable amounts of copper, and in fact liver copper accounts for at least half the copper in the whole body (Widdowson and Spray, 1951). The baby would need considerably more than the amounts provided by any of these milks, or by human milk, to maintain the concentration of copper in its body and liver while it is doubling its birthweight, even if most of the copper in the milk were absorbed. However, we know that the store of copper in the liver at birth is drawn upon during the first months afterwards, while the baby is living on milk. There is ample sufficiency of it in the liver to provide for the needs of the rest of the body during this time, and it is a matter of opinion whether it is advantageous to provide the fullterm baby with extra copper by mouth. Premature babies do not have this store of copper in the liver, and cases of hypocupraemia in premature infants fed on cows' milk have been reported (Al Rashid and Spangler, 1971).

Human milk contains enough zinc for the growing baby while it is doubling its birthweight, and cows' milk contains six times as much. Again the lowest values for zinc were found in those milks for which whey is used as the main source of protein.

VITAMINS

Measurements of the amounts of vitamins in the milks were not made. The information given on the packets or tins was sometimes helpful, but more often not. It does not seem profitable therefore to discuss this aspect of their composition.

FUTURE TRENDS

Where do the manufacturers go from here? There is no doubt that babies in Britain have flourished on preparations made from full cream cows' milk for many years. However, British firms will in all probability follow their European and American counterparts in replacing all or part of the milk fat with other fats containing more linoleic acid, and in fact they may be forced by legislation to do so. Whether they will move to the type of product made by the Dutch firm Nutricia, Almiron B, and use maize oil as the sole source of fat, besides using whey as the main source of protein, and carbohydrate other than lactose as the main source of carbohydrate, remains to be seen.

There is no evidence that sucrose, glucose or dextrimaltose are less well digested by babies than lactose, and their use will probably increase because they are cheaper than lactose. There seems no particular advantage in using whey proteins for fullterm babies, but if it is desired to reduce the amount of one or other of the inorganic constituents, the use of demineralised whey affords a method of doing this. Whether iron and copper should be added remains an open question. The Codex Committee is considering it at an administrative level. Let us hope they take into account all the relevant scientific evidence before they make their pronouncement.

One final point. How does the body fat of Dutch babies having 20 g or more of maize oil a day compare with the body fat of British babies living on full cream cows' milk?

ACKNOWLEDGEMENTS

I should like to thank Dr W. F. J. Cuthbertson and Mr A. J. Macfarlane of Glaxo Research Ltd for their help over obtaining the samples of milks, and Dr D. A. T. Southgate, Mr Y. Schutz, Mr W. Branch, Mr P. John, Mrs C. Artavanis and Miss B. Green for their contribution to the analyses.

REFERENCES

Al Rashid, R. A. and Spangler, J. (1971). *New Engl. J. Med.*, **285**, 841.
Barltrop, D. and Oppé, T. E. (1970). *Lancet*, **2**, 1333.
Bullen, J. J., Rogers, H. J. and Leigh, L. (1972). *Br. med. J.*, **1**, 69.
Gerstenberger, H. J. and Ruh, H. O. (1919). *Am. J. Dis. Child.*, **17**, 1.
Holt, L. E. Jr., Tidwell, H. C., Kirk, C. M., Cross, D. M. and Neale, S. (1935). *J. Pediat.*, **6**, 427.
Oppé, T. E. and Redstone, D. (1968). *Lancet*, **1**. 1045.
Shaw, J. C. L., Jones, A. and Gunther, M. (1973). *Br. med. J.*, **2**, 12.
Southgate, D. A. T., Widdowson, E. M., Smits, B. J., Cooke, W. T., Walker, C. H. M. and Mathers, N. P. (1969). *Lancet*, **1**, 487.
Taitz, L. S. and Byers, H. O. (1972). *Archs Dis. Childh.*, **47**, 257.
Widdowson, E. M. (1965). *Lancet*, **2**, 1099.
Widdowson, E. M. (1969). *Jl R. Coll. Phycns. Lond.*, **3**, 285.
Widdowson, E. M. and Spray, C. M. (1951). *Archs Dis. Childh.*, **26**, 205.

CHAPTER 11

Special problems of feeding very low birthweight infants

J. C. L. SHAW

Department of Paediatrics, University College Hospital Medical School, London

Malnutrition is one of the most important problems facing the very low birthweight infant; it is an inevitable consequence of premature birth and is most severe in those infants who are born most prematurely. These infants have trivial stores of body fat (Widdowson and Dickerson, 1961), glycogen (Shelley and Neligan, 1966) and trace minerals (Widdowson and Dickerson, 1961); and calculations based on their estimated energy reserves, and rate of energy expenditure have shown that they may be expected to die of starvation in about four days unless adequate nutrition is provided (Heird *et al.*, 1972). The full-term infant on the other hand has substantial stores of body fat and glycogen, and similar calculations show that he would survive starvation for a month or more. In addition to the immediate hazards there is evidence that malnutrition early in development may affect the developing brain, by permanently reducing it in both size and cell number, a state of affairs that cannot be reversed by liberal feeding later on (Ciba Foundation Symposium, 1972). Figure 1 contrasts a normal full-term infant with a low birthweight infant who is small for gestational age, and illustrates the challenge facing the paediatrician. The extreme degree of emaciation which is shown here resulted from intrauterine malnutrition, but it is not so different from the appearance of a normally developed preterm low birthweight infant. The extremely rapid rate of growth of these infants, and their trivial body stores makes the provision of adequate nutrition an urgent matter.

The ideal dietary allowance of different substances for a full-term infant may be inferred from the known composition of breast milk and the volumes of milk ingested by normal infants. But it would be wrong to assume that allowances thus calculated would necessarily be suitable for low birthweight preterm infants.

The ideal nutrition of the low birthweight preterm infant should be such that his postnatal growth is both quantitatively and qualitatively similar to that, that would have occurred, had he remained *in utero*, so it is to intrauterine growth that we should turn for information on the proper nutrition of the low birthweight infant. Figure 2 compares two

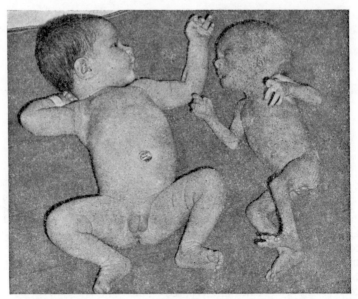

Fig. 1. *Comparison of a full-term 3·5 kg infant with an infant of 37 weeks gestation whose birthweight was 1·3 kg, more than 700 g below the 10th percentile for gestational age.*

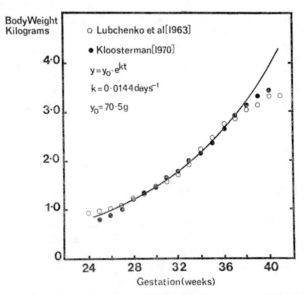

Fig. 2. *Comparison of the mean values for birthweight of infants born at different periods of gestation from the data of Lubchenko et al. (1963) and Kloosterman (1970). Weight gain between 24 and 36 weeks is exponential in character.*

intrauterine growth curves obtained from the mean values for birthweight, of infants born at different periods of gestation. The data of Kloosterman (1970) were from infants born at sea level whereas those of Lubchenko et al. (1963) were from infants born in Denver, Colorado, one mile above sea level. It can be seen that between 24 and 36 weeks gestation growth *in*

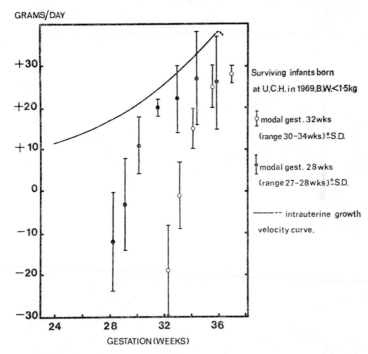

Fig. 3. Comparison of calculated intrauterine growth velocity with the measured growth rate of all the infants born in University College Hospital in 1969 and weighing less than 1·5 kg. Only in exceptional cases did the growth of these infants exceed intrauterine growth rate.

utero can be described by the exponential equation $Y = Y_0 \cdot e^{kt}$† and| occurs at a rate of 1·44%/day. Using this rate constant (k) the growth velocity at different periods of gestation can be calculated and a growth velocity curve constructed. Figure 3 compares this intrauterine

† Mathematical methods. The regression lines in Figs. 2 and 4 were fitted to the data by the method of least squares using the exponential equation $Y = Y_0 \cdot e^{kt}$. Y is the value on the Y axis at time t, and Y_0 is the value of Y when $t = 0$. k is a rate constant and the slope of the regression line (dY/dt) at any point is given by the expression $k \times Y$.

118

J. C. L. SHAW

growth velocity curve with the postnatal growth rate of two groups of infants of birthweight less than 1·5 kg. It can be seen that only exceptionally did postnatal growth rate equal or exceed intrauterine growth rate, and this represents a substantial degree of malnutrition.

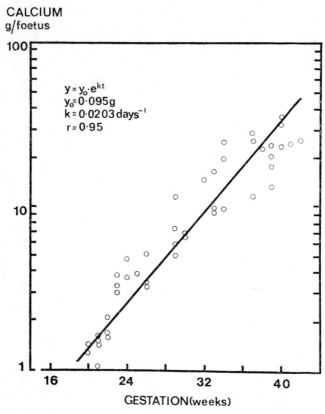

Fig. 4. Results of analyses of foetal bodies for calcium (Kelly et al., 1950; Widdowson and Dickerson, 1961). The accumulation of calcium by the foetus between 26 and 40 weeks can be adequately described by a simple exponential equation.

Just as weight gain is exponential between 28 and 36 weeks gestation, so is the accumulation of different elements. Figure 4 gives, as an example, the results of the analyses of foetal bodies for calcium performed over the last 80 years (Widdowson and Dickerson, 1961; Kelly *et al.*, 1950). The accumulation of calcium by the human foetus between 20 and 40 weeks gestation can also be adequately described by the exponential equation $Y = Y_0 \cdot e^{kt}$ and it can be calculated that calcium accumulates at a rate of 2·03%/day. Figure 5 gives the results of similar calculations using all the available data from the analyses of foetal bodies, and provides a reference standard for the nutrition of low birthweight infants. It can be seen that the rate constants for all elements are very similar, with the notable exception of fat which is laid down extremely rapidly in the last few weeks of pregnancy. Apart from their obvious value in evaluating the

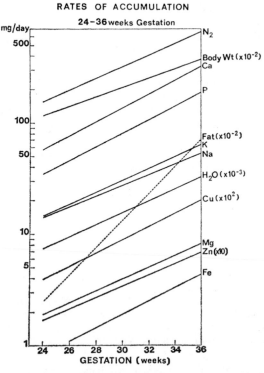

Fig. 5. *The calculated rates of accumulation of different substances by the human foetus between 24 and 36 weeks gestation.*

dietary intake of different substances these calculated rates of accumulation can be compared directly with the measured retentions of different elements in post-natal life, and this gives us a valuable tool with which to investigate the adequacy or otherwise of different diets.

I have been studying the absorption and retention of calcium in low birthweight infants because it became apparent that human breast milk, since it has so little calcium in it, could never meet the calcium requirements of these infants; and, because calcium is only partly absorbed it seemed possible that even cows' milk would not provide an adequate amount of calcium for these infants. The data I am presenting today is from a study of ten low birthweight infants of 28–31 weeks gestation and of birthweight 1110–1390 g. They have been studied by metabolic balance techniques continuously for periods of 20–60 days. The metabolic balances commence on day 10 where possible, and a balance was performed every 5 days until the child is discharged home between the 60th and 70th day of life. Aliquots of diet and stool were analysed for calcium and fat; calcium by flame photometry and fat by the method of van de Kamer et al. (1949). Complete 24-hour urine collections were made every 5 days in order to estimate the loss of calcium in the urine. This urinary loss of calcium was at all times a small amount, and could have been safely ignored. The infants were fed on four diets; a full cream cows' milk, a half skimmed cows' milk, SMA and breast milk. The composition of the milks is shown in Table 1. The two cows' milk diets were selected to see if altering the fat content made any difference to the amount of calcium absorbed. All infants received 25 μg of cholecalciferol daily from day 7.

TABLE 1

COMPOSITION OF MILKS

Milk	Ca (Mean $\pm$ SD) (g/litre)	Fat[a] (g/litre)
Half cream cows' milk ($n = 6$)	$1\cdot028 \pm 0\cdot047$	$14\cdot0 \pm 1\cdot0$
Full cream cows' milk ($n = 7$)	$1\cdot054 \pm 0\cdot057$	$28\cdot0 \pm 3\cdot0$
SMA	$0\cdot623 \pm 0\cdot063$	$29\cdot0 \pm 2\cdot0$
Breast milk	$0\cdot285 \pm 0\cdot026$	$26\cdot0 \pm 4\cdot0$

[a] Fats measured by method of van de Kamer et al. (1949).

Measurements of fat absorption confirmed what is already known (Tidwell et al., 1935); that premature infants malabsorb fat to a serious degree. Figure 6 summarises the results of the fat balances. The fat of breast milk was the most completely absorbed (85% $\pm$ 1·8 SE). The proportion of fat absorbed, from half cream cows' milk (60% $\pm$ 1·9 SE) and SMA (62% $\pm$ 1·7 SE) were not significantly different but when cows' milk fat was fed in full amounts the absorption was very much reduced (46% $\pm$ 2·3 SE). Most important in these studies is the fact that there seems to be little if any improvement in the proportion of fat absorbed in premature infants between the 10th and the 70th day of life.

Figure 7 compares the measured retentions of calcium in two infants on different milks, with the range of intrauterine calcium accumulation to be

FAT ABSORPTION
g/kg.day

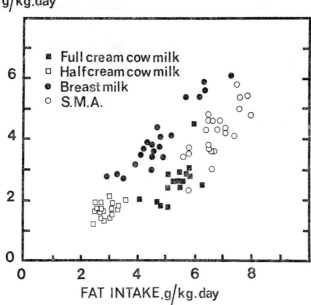

Fig. 6. Results of fat balances. The absorption of fat from breast milk was 85% (±1·8 SE), from SMA 62% (±1·7 SE), from half cream cows' milk 60% (±1·9 SE) and from full cream cows' milk 46% (±2·3 SE).

TABLE 2

COMPARISON OF MEASURED CALCIUM RETENTION IN TEN PREMATURE INFANTS BETWEEN THE 10TH AND 70TH DAY OF LIFE, WITH ESTIMATED ACCUMULATION OF CALCIUM BY THE HUMAN FOETUS OVER AN EQUIVALENT PERIOD *in utero*

Milk	No. of infants	Duration of balance (days)	Total calcium retained (g ± SD)	Estimated intrauterine accumulation (g)	Retention as a % of intrauterine accumulation
Half cream cows' milk	3	20–50	5·4 ± 2·9	15·4	35
Full cream cows' milk	2	60	6·4 ± 0·3	21·1	30
SMA	3	45–60	3·6 ± 1·2	19·9	18
Breast milk	2	52–60	3·3 ± 0·4	19·4	17

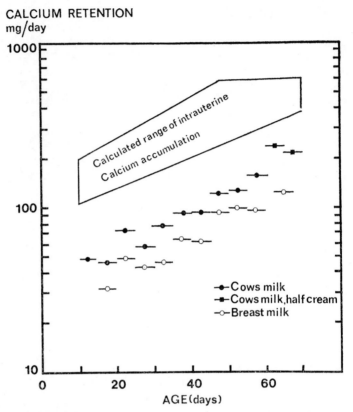

Fig. 7. *Comparison of calcium balances of two infants fed different milks, with the range of intrauterine calcium accumulation to be expected in the infants under study.*

expected in the infants under study. The infant fed cows' milk absorbed more calcium than the infant fed breast milk, but even so both these infants and all the others studied developed a gross deficit in body calcium by the time they were discharged home. Table 2 summarises the results of the calcium balances and shows the effect of halving the dietary fat on the amount of calcium absorbed. The retention of calcium by infants fed cows' milk was about a third only of the estimated intrauterine accumulation over an equivalent period *in utero*, and the differences attributable to the different fat content were small, and not statistically significant. The retentions of calcium by infants fed SMA and breast milk were less than a fifth of that they would have accumulated had they remained *in utero*. It is worth pointing out here that the inevitable errors inherent in metabolic balances are not self-cancelling but are additive and tend to overestimate the amount of a substance retained in the body. The body deficit, therefore, in these infants is probably greater than would appear from these data (Wallace, 1959). These results raise serious questions. Are there for instance, deficits of other nutrients of similar magnitude? Nitrogen is the only other element that has been extensively studied by metabolic balance techniques (Snyderman et al., 1969), and the results though confusing do show that nitrogen is readily absorbed and that body deficits of the magnitude observed with calcium probably do not occur. We are currently investigating the absorption and retention of trace elements because from our knowledge of the rate at which some of them accumulate *in utero* it seems likely that deficiencies may arise. An equally important question concerns what we should do to improve the absorption of calcium and fat. One promising approach is to feed a high calcium milk such as cows' milk with the fat replaced by medium chain triglycerides and a small amount of vegetable oil such as maize oil to supply the essential fatty acids. A preliminary report of such diets used in low birthweight infants are very encouraging (Tantibhedhyangkul and Hashin, 1971).

CONCLUSIONS

Using the growth of the foetus *in utero* as a standard of reference, it becomes clear that the nutritional requirements of low birthweight infants are in many instances quite different from those of full-term infants and this suggests that a specialised product may indeed be required to feed these infants. Breast milk while undeniably deficient in calcium has nonetheless characteristics that recommend its use. The fat is well absorbed by low birthweight infants and the presence of such substances as lactoferrin (Bullen et al., 1972) and immunoglobulins may have an important bearing on the health and nutrition of these infants. The deficient skeletal mineralisation has yet to be proved harmful and may be ameliorated by increasing the volume of feed to 300 ml/kg/day (Valman et al., 1972). For these reasons I think it would be wrong to say that breast milk is unsuitable for low birthweight infants, and in underdeveloped countries it is still the food of choice. However, the difficulty of securing adequate supplies of breast milk in this country has meant that most newborn units use a preparation based on cows' milk and it seems unlikely that this situation will change in the near future. The milk preparations I have used in the investigations reported here, are representative of those used elsewhere in Britain and none seem entirely satisfactory. It therefore seems certain that as we learn more about the nutritional requirements and absorptive capacity of these infants, there will be plenty of scope for developing a milk food adapted to the special needs of very low birthweight infants.

124 J. C. L. SHAW

REFERENCES

Bullen, J. J., Rogers, H. J. and Leigh, L. (1972). *Br. med. J.*, **1,** 69.
Ciba Foundation Symposium (1972). *Lipids, Malnutrition and the Developing Brain* (with the Nestlé Foundation), edited by K. Elliott and J. Knight Associated Scientific Publishers, Amsterdam, London, New York.
Heird, W. C., Driscoll, J. M., Jr., Schullinger, J. N., Grebin, B. and Winters, R. W. (1972). *J. Pediat.*, **80,** 351.
Kelly, H. J., Sloan, R. E., Hoffman, W. and Saunders, C. (1950). 'Accumulation of nitrogen and six minerals in the human foetus during gestation', *Hum. Biol.*, **2,** 61.
Kloosterman, G. J. (1970). *Int. J. Gynec. and Obstet.*, **8,** 895.
Lubchenko, L. O., Hansman, C., Dressler, M. and Boyd, E. (1963). *Pediatrics, Springfield*, **32,** 793.
Shelley, H. J. and Neligan, G. A. (1966). *Br. med. Bull.*, **22,** 34.
Snyderman, S. E., Boyer, A., Kogut, M. D. and Holt, L. E., Jr. (1969). *J. Pediat.*, **74,** 874.
Tantibhedhyangkul, P. and Hashin, S. A. (1971). *Bull. N.Y. Acad. Med.*, **47,** 17.
Tidwell, H. C., Holt, L. E., Jr., Farrow, H. L. and Neale, S. (1935).*J. Pediat.*, **6,** 481.
Valman, H. B., Heath, C. D. and Brown, R. K. J. (1972)., *Br. med. J.*, **3,** 547.
van de Kamer, J. H., ten Bokkel Huinink, H. and Weijers, H. A. (1949). 'Rapid method for the determination of fat in faeces', *J. biol. Chem.*, **177,** 347.
Wallace, W. M. (1959). *Fedn Proc.*, **18,** 1125.
Widdowson, E. M. and Dickerson, J. W. T. (1961). In *Mineral Metabolism*, edited by C. L. Comar and F. Bronner, Vol. II, part A, Academic Press, New York and London.

CHAPTER 12

Possible effects of incorrectly prepared formulae on weight gain and electrolyte disturbances in infants

L. S. TAITZ

The Children's Hospital, Sheffield

In recent years, certain trends in the feeding of young infants have emerged which are in many ways a direct counterpart of certain developments in society generally. These may best be described as the outcome of two major dogmas of our age, that restrictions and disciplines of any kind are suspect, and that technological innovation can automatically resolve the difficulties inherent in the abandonment of natural processes in favour of artificial ones (Taitz, 1972). The great danger of this climate of opinion has always been that we are all too ready to adopt new methods without showing either that they are intrinsically better than the old, or, even worse, that they are fundamentally safe either in the short or the long term. Infant nutrition has been peculiarly susceptible to these trends, and only very recently have serious questions begun to be asked about the desirability of the virtual disappearance of breast feeding coupled with the fashion for very early introduction of non-milk feeds into the diets of very young infants.

It is the aim of this communication to draw attention to some potential dangers of these tendencies and to point out, at the very least, the need to demonstrate that they are harmless.

FACTORS WHICH CONTROL DIETARY INTAKE

There has been an assumption underlying much advice on infant feeding which requires serious challenge, namely that it is 'impossible to overfeed an infant'. This notion almost certainly arises from the fact that babies tend to adjust their volume of intake to the energy content of the diet (Ziegler and Fomon, 1971). Babies who are breast fed tend to take enough milk to supply the average requirement of 100 kcal (418 kJ)/kg/day. Since milk provides about 110 kcal (460 kJ)/150 ml, the latter value represents the average fluid intake of breast-fed infants. The basal water requirement is 100 ml/kg/day. Infants therefore have an excess water intake and it is tempting to assume that this is an evolutionary safety valve for all those sudden switches of external water balance to which infants are both prey and dangerously vulnerable.

The second mechanism which may influence the volume of intake is the thirst impulse. Babies in external water deficit would be expected to have some elevation of extracellular osmolality which in the first instance produces sensation of thirst and in the second leads to a reduction of urinary volume, reducing water loss on the one hand and on the other leading to an increased intake as the mother responds to the insistent demand. These processes depend for their efficacy on the ability of the mother to recognise the distinction between hunger and thirst and the capacity of the infant kidney to conserve water. Any survey will show that the first condition is often not met and that the general response to a crying baby is the assumption of hunger rather than thirst.

The question of urinary concentrating power is complicated. Edelman and Barnett (1960) have shown that infants are capable of attaining maximal urinary osmolalities in the range of the adult kidney. Our own studies confirm the suggestion that the main factor deciding the concentration of the urine is the solute load in the diet (Table 1). The breast-fed infants

TABLE 1

URINARY SOLUTE AND OSMOLAR CONCENTRATIONS IN
INFANTS AGED 6 TO 10 WEEKS

(Mean concentrations of random urine samples)

	Urea concentration (mg/100 ml)	Osmolar concentration (mOsm/kg)	Number of samples
Breast fed (low solute feed)	211·4	104·6	19
Cows' milk (high solute feed)	1007·3	377·9	15

showed average *random* osmolalities which were three times lower than those of artificially fed infants. Although infants are capable of considerable feats of urine concentration, it does not follow that the administration of high solute loads is desirable or even safe. One possible ill effect of this is illustrated in the following argument.

THE SOLUTE LOAD OF ARTIFICIAL FEEDING

The solute load imposed by cows' milk formula is much higher than that of breast milk. Two main factors are responsible for this—the high sodium content of cows' milk (23 mEq/litre) as opposed to breast milk (7 mEq/litre) and the fact that much of the energy source from cows' milk consists of keto acids from the amino acids present in excess in the diets of cows' milk fed babies. The deamination of these amino acids produces a large quantity of urea. This is illustrated in the data in Table 1. It is also reflected in the high urinary osmolar concentrations referred to in the previous section. It is important to consider these high solute loads in relation to the total water intake and the energy intake.

Cows' milk has the same energy value as human milk. Thus the intake of water in cows' milk fed babies can be expected to be identical to that of breast-fed babies. However, the obligatory urinary water excretion is much higher in artificially fed infants because the solute load is so much greater. If a breast-fed infant increases his insensible water loss for any reason such as overheating or hyperventilation, or has an episode of diarrhoea or loses fluid through a weeping skin rash, the work required of the kidney in reducing urinary water loss is much smaller than that of an infant fed cows' milk. One would therefore expect, on theoretical grounds, that breast-fed infants would be less susceptible to dehydration and hypernatraemia than artificially fed babies.

THE EFFECTS OF INCORRECT FEEDING PRACTICES

Recent studies have indicated that there is a wide margin of error in the preparation of infant feed from the powdered preparation (Taitz and Byers, 1972). Our data show that a high proportion of milk feeds bought by mothers coming to the well-baby follow-up clinic contain too much milk powder (Table 2). In some cases the error is gross, bringing the sodium

TABLE 2

SODIUM CONCENTRATIONS OF MILK FEEDS PREPARED
BY MOTHERS

	Sodium concentrations		
	<30 mEq/litre	30–35 mEq/litre	>35 mEq/litre
Number	11	14	6

concentration of the feed into the range which has previously been shown to precipitate hypertonic dehydration in infants with diarrhoea (Colle *et al.*, 1958). The effect of high solute feeds on the incidence of hypernatraemia is now well recognised and may be due to the administration of concentrated skimmed milk or formula boiled after preparation (Berenberg *et al.*, 1969; Finberg, 1969).

The possible errors of measurement which result in the incorrectly prepared formula are many. They result from the fact that mothers either ignore the instructions on the package, or misinterpret them, or claim to have been incorrectly advised. The following is a list of some of the mistakes which are made:

1. packing down the powder instead of scraping it off the scoop with a knife;
2. scraping the scoop against the side of the packet;
3. not bothering to count the scoops or losing count;
4. using heaped scoops;
5. deliberately using extra scoops.

It is interesting that mothers often regard these questions with some amusement and seem surprised that they should be considered important.

It can therefore be stated with some confidence that lack of care in the preparation of milk feeds is commonplace and that this leads to significant errors in the composition of the feeds.

This tendency to prepare overconcentrated feeds has two obvious effects. It increases the ratio of both solute and energy to that of water intake. The hunger of the infants will then be sated by a smaller total volume. This reduction of water intake has several potentially harmful effects. In the first instance it reduces the margin of safety imparted by the delicate balance which supplies adequate energy in an excess of water. The consequences of a reduction of intake of the order suggested by the sodium composition found in our sample is illustrated in Table 3, which shows

TABLE 3

POSSIBLE EFFECT ON URINE VOLUME OF 20% EXCESS IN CONCENTRATION OF FEEDS

	Energy content in 150 ml (kJ)	Volume required for adequate energy intake (ml/kg/24 hours)	Insensible loss (ml/kg/24 hours)	Urine volume (ml/kg/24 hours)
Correctly prepared	460	150	50	100
Overconcentrated	552	125	50	75

that the possible urinary volume is reduced by 25% while the solute load is considerably increased. A sudden increase in non-urinary water losses would gravely embarrass the overall water economy of such infants.

The need to excrete a large solute load with a decreased water intake may also account for the fact that many artificially fed babies are difficult to satisfy. The failure of mothers to distinguish between hunger and thirst may lead to progressively rising intakes of concentrated feed, giving way at last to the introduction of solid foods. This factor may account for the tendency for babies to be offered solids early, thus compounding the problem of high solute to water and high energy to water ratios, especially as many baby foods are high in salt and even make a virtue of containing protein additives, which increase solute load. The practice of crumbling rusks into milk feeds is typical of the tendency to alter the delicate natural balance of unadulterated milk.

POSSIBLE DANGERS OF HIGH SOLUTE/ENERGY FEEDING

Excess weight gain

Most workers agree that artificially fed babies gain weight faster than breast-fed infants in the first weeks of life (Baum, 1971; Tracey et al., 1971; Taitz, 1971). This tendency appears to be due not so much to the type of feeding but to errors and practices associated with it. If infants who are artificially fed were to be restricted to the 110 kcal (460 kJ)/150 ml of fluid no doubt the phenomenon would not occur and it is possible that, in those studies which do not show it, the results are influenced by the unusually excellent medical advice (Adebonojo, 1972). The apparent tendency for artificially fed infants to gain weight faster than those who are breast fed is illustrated in Table 4, by comparing the data of Fomon and

TABLE 4

90TH CENTILE FOR WEIGHT—6 WEEKS

	Males	Females
Fomon and Filer (1970) (breast fed only)	5·35	4·7
Tanner and Whitehouse (1959)	5·45	5·05
Tanner et al. (1966)	5·50	5·1
Taitz and Harris (1972) (artificial feeds only)	5·75	5·4

Filer and those from Sheffield. The apparent continuing trend for weights to increase in Britain is also of interest (Fomon and Filer, 1970; Taitz and Harris, 1972; Tanner et al., 1966), in view of the continued trend away from breast feeding and towards the early introduction of solids. The figures for weight velocities in Sheffield, illustrated in Table 5, show how the rate of weight gain has increased during the last decade, from values close to those of a breast fed group. The real question is whether this trend is harmful or not. The potential danger lies in the suggestion that rapid

TABLE 5

WEIGHT VELOCITIES AT SIX WEEKS
(g/day)

	Males			Females		
	10th Centile	50th Centile	90th Centile	10th Centile	50th Centile	90th Centile
Fomon and Filer (1970) (breast-fed infants)	18·7	30·8	43·3	18·5	27·3	34·7
Eid (1970) (Sheffield children born in 1961)	18·9	27·1	36·5	17·6	25·7	35·8
Taitz and Harris (1972) (Sheffield children born in 1972)	28·0	35·6	51·0	26·0	34·7	43·0

weight gain in early infancy may predispose to childhood obesity (Anonymous, 1970), and therefore to adult obesity with all the undoubted harmful effects of that state (Mullins, 1958; Lloyd et al., 1961). Eid (1970) has shown that babies with excessive neonatal weight gain have about four times the risk of childhood obesity when compared with infants who do not show excessive early weight gain, possibly by determining the number of adipose cells in later life (Beaton, 1967). It would be prudent to assume that high energy diets due to concentrated feeds and early introduction of solids are not the ideal feeding practice.

Danger of hypertonic dehydration

Hypertonic dehydration rarely occurs in breast-fed babies and it is clear that gross feeding preparation errors are an important factor in the pathogenesis of the condition (Skinner, 1967; Stern et al., 1972). Only recently attention has been drawn to the possibility that smaller but persistent mistakes may place the infant at risk. There is certainly a case for greater care in preparation of formulae. It may even be worth asking whether the present practice of allowing a greater proportion of energy to be derived from protein with a relative reduction in sugar content is the best solution. Perhaps it might be safer to assume considerable error in measurement and to reduce the milk powder correspondingly.

The possible dangers of high sodium intake in early infancy

There has recently been considerable controversy in the US regarding the high sodium content of some baby foods (Filer, 1971). This has been criticised because of experimental evidence that sodium loading may cause hypertension (Dahl et al., 1962). Others have defended the manufacturers on the grounds that there is no convincing proof that this may be true of humans (Lowe, 1972). Not only do some foods contain high sodium contents, but in using full strength cows' milk we are already offering infants a salt intake about four times greater than that which nature apparently intended. If our observation that many feeds are too concentrated is correct, then the salt content is often even higher than this. It is impossible not to be concerned about this, even in the absence of absolute evidence of possible harm. It seems reasonable to assume that when the composition of a young infant's diet is radically different from that of breast milk some trouble is to be expected. Any deviation from the food which has been evolved by a slow evolutionary process must surely be viewed with suspicion. The onus of proof must be on those who seek to show that such deviations are desirable *and* safe, and not the other way round. It is difficult in the circumstances to disagree with the dictum recently enunciated by Gellis (1972) that 'Human milk is for babies, and cows' milk is for calves'.

SUMMARY

1. The factors which control the dietary intakes of young infants are complex, comprising a delicate balance of energy, solute and water, which may easily be upset.
2. The possible harmful effects of such resulting imbalances are discussed with special reference to obesity, hypertonic dehydration and hypertension.
3. It can safely be concluded that breast feeding remains the optimal dietary regime for young babies and that the burden of proof that innovations, such as early weaning, high sodium intakes and high solute/water ratios are safe, lies on those who suggest or defend them.

REFERENCES

Adebonojo, F. O. (1972). *Clin. Pediat.*, **11**, 25.

Anonymous (1970). *Br. med. J.*, **2**, 64.

Baum, J. D. (1971). *Obstet. and Gynec.*, **37**, 126.

Beaton, J. R. (1967). *Can. J. publ. Hlth.*, **58**, 479.

Berenberg, W., Mendell, F. and Fellers, F. X. (1969). *Pediatrics, Springfield*, **44**, 734.

Colle, E., Ayoub, E. and Raile, R. (1958). *Pediatrics, Springfield*, **22**, 5.

Dahl, L. K., Heine, M. and Tassinari, L. E. (1962). *J. exp. Med.*, **115**, 1173.

Edelman, C. M., Jr., and Barnett, H. L. (1960). *J. Pediat.*, **56**, 154.

Eid, E. E. (1970). *Br. med. J.*, **2**, 74.

Filer, I. J. (1971). *Nutr. Rev.*, **29**, 27.

Finberg, L. (1969). 'Hypernatraemia in Infants as cause of Brain Damage'. In *Year Book of Pediatrics*, p. 49. Year Book Medical Publishers, Chicago.

Fomon, S. J. and Filer, L. J. (1970). *Acta paediat., Stockh.*, **Supp. 202**, p. 1.

Gellis, S. S. (1972). Footnote in *Year Book of Pediatrics*, p. 21. Year Book Medical Publishers, Chicago.

Lloyd, J. K., Wolff, O. H. and Whelan, M. S. (1961). *Br. med. J.*, **2**, 145.

Lowe, C. U. (1972). *Am. J. clin. Nutr.*, **25**, 245.

Mullins, A. G. (1958). *Archs Dis. Childh.*, **33**, 307.

Skinner, A. L. (1967). *Pediatrics, Springfield*, **39**, 625.

Stern, G. M., Jones, R. B. and Fraser, A. C. L. (1972). *Archs Dis. Childh.*, **47**, 468.

Taitz, L. S. (1971). *Br. med. J.*, **1**, 315.

Taitz, L. S. (1972). *Nutrition, Lond.*, **26**, 339.

Taitz, L. S. and Byers, H. D. (1972). *Archs Dis. Childh.*, **47**, 257.

Taitz, L. S. and Harris, F. (1972). Unpublished data.

Tanner, J. M. and Whitehouse, R. H. (1959). *Height and Weight Standard Charts*, Institute of Child Health, London.

Tanner, J. M., Whitehouse, R. H. and Takaishi, M. (1966). *Archs Dis. Childh.*, **41**, 613.

Tracey, V. V., De, N. C. and Harper, J. R. (1971). *Br. med. J.*, **1**, 16.

Ziegler, E. E. and Fomon, S. J. (1971). *J. Pediat.*, **78**, 561.

PART 3

THE NATIONAL CHILD DEVELOPMENT SURVEY

CHAPTER 13

Some nutritional aspects of large scale prospective studies in child development

EUAN M. ROSS

Department of Child Health, Royal Hospital for Sick Children, Bristol

It may seem out of place that two consecutive papers are being presented at a conference of the British Nutrition Foundation based on a study where the nature of diet consumed was at no time assayed. It is difficult enough to study the dietary habits of even the lowliest of animals under controlled conditions, and the enormous difficulties of such studies on humans is the reason why conferences of this nature are required. Much of our knowledge of human nutrition is based on informed observations made when man inadvertently places himself under experimental conditions, such as war. Physician to the Fleet Dr James Lind (1753), who discovered the anti-scorbutic properties of oranges and lemons, was an early example. More recently Dicke's finding that gluten was the noxious factor in coeliac disease during the 1939–45 War serves as another illustration (Dicke *et al.*, 1953). What can we do in times of peace? My role is to be prologue to the distinguished colleagues who have methodically studied the fate of 17 000 pregnancies and in so doing learned a great deal about the ways in which our nation's children grow up. I shall later deal with some findings from a large scale study in which I have had the honour of participation. But it is first necessary to say something about prospective studies of large populations and their role in monitoring the health of nations.

Individual prospective studies of child development have been carried out for generations by proud parents who have measured their offspring. The first such study to reach the medical literature was performed by de Montbeillard (cited by Scammon, 1927) on his son during the period 1759–77. Not long afterwards in 1787 Tiedemann (cited by Murchison and Larger, 1927) described the serial psychomotor development of his son. Charles Darwin (1877) similarly studied his family.

The first longitudinal growth study of a series of individuals appears to have been carried out in Vienna in the mid-19th century (Liharzik, 1858). His results formed the basis of the first tables of child height and weight. From simple beginnings in which local groups of children were documented mainly from a physical standpoint, came the realisation that such studies must be based on sound statistical principles, an example being the studies of Sir Cyril Burt (1937) whose works on London school-children are now of classical interest.

Throughout the past 25 years, expertise in the conduct of large scale studies has been gradually built up, both in the United Kingdom and elsewhere. The possibilities and, all too often, the limitations of such studies are gradually becoming recognised.

The major early postwar British studies of Spence (Spence *et al.*, 1954) on the Newcastle 1000 families and James Douglas's cohort study starting in 1947 (Douglas and Blomfield, 1958) did a great deal to speed up social change in this country and exert a continuing influence on subsequent studies.

A detailed review of longitudinal studies in child development carried out throughout the world is being compiled by Zachau-Christiansen and Ross (in press) with a view to publication next year.

Large scale longitudinal studies involving many thousands of individuals, however, cannot undertake actual analysis of the diet of mothers in pregnancy and their influence on the foetus. Thus they add little to the important matters so freely discussed in our Sunday papers such as the consumption of blighted potatoes, hardness of water, fluoride content, tea, coffee, refined sugar and vitamin content of the diet and their relationship to foetal malformation and possible influence on the health of infants. It is, however, possible to undertake indirect studies of nutrition. Certain aspects of human life are relatively easy to document. For example, where one lives, type of housing, work, rest and health in its many aspects can be gathered and contrasted with the weight and height of offspring and parents.

I wish now to return to findings from the National Child Development Study—1958 Cohort (NCDS) involving the births in England, Scotland and Wales in the period 3–9th March 1958. During this period, a Perinatal Mortality Study was held in which data were collected on all births (bar a 2% loss) occurring during this week. Midwives attending mothers were asked to fill in precoded questionnaires containing details of mother's health, social background, marital arrangements, employment in pregnancy and use of antenatal services. The course and conduct of the pregnancy and delivery was studied, and the health of the ensuing foetus recorded. In order to be able to make meaningful comparisons between successful and unsuccessful pregnancies, all stillbirths and first week deaths occurring during the following three months were also scrutinised and postmortem studies carried out wherever possible. This work took place whilst I was still a medical student, and the story rightly belongs to Neville Butler, to whom is due the credit for organising and inspiring such an extraordinary study. The results of this study have been published (Butler and Bonham (1963); Butler and Alberman (1969); further papers are still appearing).

With Government funding it became possible to study surviving children in 1965, when, as a result of a massive tracing and testing exercise, 15 500 survivors (92 % of the original sample) were found. This sample is known as the National Child Development Study. The parents were interviewed at home by health visitors. Detailed medical examinations on these children were carried out at schools and teachers were also asked to perform a series of educational tests and assessments. Again, it was not possible to study the content of diets of these seven-year-old children on a national scale, but questions concerning feeding patterns in infancy and current appetite were asked. Children were weighed and measured by methods suggested by Tanner (1962).

Some of the results of this study have been published by Davie et al. (1972) and others. Follow-up studies of these children were repeated in 1969 when the children were aged 11 when a similar exercise was carried out—again with a gratifyingly high response rate. A further comprehensive follow-up is intended for autumn 1973 before children leave school. It is hoped that it will be possible to continue the study into adult life.

What of results? At the last count we possessed 2×10^7 individual facts about these children (Goldstein, 1973). I shall now concentrate on some aspects relevant to this meeting.

NUTRITIONAL INFLUENCES ON THE FOETUS

The size of an infant at birth represents a summation of many factors. Studies by Ounsted and Ounsted (1973) show that a mother's own size has a subtle constraint on the birthweight of her children. Their findings supplement those made long ago by Hammond who crossed Shetland ponies with Shire horses and produced a series of hybrid nags. Shetland mothers have Shetland size foals even if father is four times her size. We now well realise that the foetus is not a parasite who indiscriminately abstracts food from the mother. As an illustration, Pakistani mothers tend to have larger babies in Britain than in their homeland. The NCDS shows quite marked differences in the proportion of low birthweight babies in the different social classes. This is particularly the case in babies of unmarried mothers of whom no less than 11 % had low weight (2500 g) babies (Crellin et al., 1971). The unmarried are known to have considerably lower spending power than the married, and hence spend less on food. These mothers were less likely to use antenatal services. Maternal anxiety, too, has a role in determining the outcome of pregnancy and hence birthweight. The unmarried have much to be anxious about (Barrett, 1971). The less well-to-do are more likely to have light-for-dates babies. These are the very mothers who tend to use antenatal services the least yet get the most antenatal complications. Perhaps the most urgent problem in foetal nutrition is smoking in pregnancy. Our study once again confirms findings consistently reported by over 20 papers since Simpson (1957) from (appropriately) the College of Medical Evangelists first showed that mothers who smoked in pregnancy had lighter babies than mothers who did not smoke. In our study there was a mean deficit in birthweight of 170 g for the latter weeks of pregnancy though gestation was not appreciably shortened. The question remains—is there a fundamental difference in life style between smokers and non-smokers causing the weight deficit rather than a true smoking effect. We investigated this question by means of a statistical counterpart to the famous confrontation of Jehovah and Baal. The data show that even when allowance is made for the fact that smoking mothers as a group are older, have larger families and are of lower average social class, their babies still weigh light. Even a recent cautious *British Medical Journal* editorial (Anonymous, 1973) begins 'No reasonable doubt now remains that smoking in pregnancy has adverse effects on the developing foetus'. Cole *et al.* (1972) found that the carbon monoxide level in the blood of the smoking mother was three times that of non-smokers and twice normal in the foetus. There have been conflicting reports on whether smoking in pregnancy actually harms the foetus. Some studies on relatively well-to-do populations—for example those of Yerushalmy (1964; 1971) on white mothers and of Rantakallio (1969) on a series of prosperous Finns—have shown smoking to have no influence on perinatal mortality. On the other hand, from the present study Butler *et al.* (1972) reported a 30% increase in perinatal mortality in the offspring of mothers who smoked in pregnancy, an effect which was still seen when like for like populations were studied where the only known difference in mothers was the fact that they did or did not smoke. A similar, though smaller, excess in perinatal mortality was reported by Andrews and McGarry (1972) from South Wales in a recently reported population study. The excess perinatal death rate appears to be due directly to the fact that the babies of smokers were proportionately smaller-for-dates than those of non-smokers. Postmortem findings showed a normal spectrum of pathology in such infants. Fedrick *et al.* (1971) later from the same sample and survivors has shown a small increase in congenital heart defects significant even after allowance for maternal age and social class. The *BMJ* editorial (Anonymous, 1973) states that there appears to be some conflict of opinion on the question whether the offspring of mothers who smoke in pregnancy show any evidence of intellectual handicap. There is not time to discuss the matter in detail, but at seven years children in the NCDS whose mothers smoked after the fourth month of pregnancy showed an average five months' retardation in reading age and were slightly shorter compared with the children of non-smokers, a trend that held true even when allowance was made for differences in social and environmental factors between the two sorts of mother.

As an example of a factor that can be studied in large scale longitudinal surveys I turn briefly to breast feeding. Paediatricians as a breed believe 'that it is a good thing' and confidently recommend it in their lectures to succeeding generations of students. Mothers, however, become even more ready to bottle feed infants and let their infants pay not even the briefest lip service to our beliefs. Earlier papers given today help to support these contentions. Approximately 31 % of infants in 1958 never tasted mother's milk. Which mothers breast feed? We found that this was practised more frequently by women of high social class, who had small families, and was most likely in the south of England. Scots mothers were particularly unlikely to breast feed—even the wives of skilled workers and professionals.

What becomes of the breast-fed babies? Do they grow up to be well adjusted, slim, coronary free, delightful individuals? Do their cows' milk fed peers degenerate early into some bovine equivalent of the centaur, half man, half cow? The NCDS promises to give us some more information about this as the years go by. We hope that our successors will study the coronary heart diseases of the study children as they occur. Already there is some evidence that children who were breast fed are less obese at 11 years old.

ACKNOWLEDGEMENT

Material contained in this paper is published by kind permission of the co-directors of the National Child Development Study. The information was gathered through the generous cooperation of parents, teachers, health visitors and medical officers of health throughout the country.

REFERENCES

Andrews, J. and McGarry, J. M. (1972). *J. Obstet. Gynaec. Br. Commonw.*, **79**, 1057.

Anonymous (1973). *Br. med. J.*, **1**, 369.

Barrett, J. (1971). In *Antenatal Paediatrics*, edited by G. F. Batstone, A. W. Blair and J. Slater, Medical and Technical Publications, Aylesbury.

Burt, C. L. (1937). *The Backward Child*, University of London Press, London.

Butler, N. R. and Alberman, E. (1969). *Perinatal Problems*, Livingstone, Edinburgh.

Butler, N. R. and Bonham, D. (1963). *Perinatal Mortality*, Livingstone, Edinburgh.

Butler, N. R., Goldstein, H. and Ross, E. M. (1972). *Br. med. J.*, **2**, 127.

Cole, P. V., Hawkins, L. M. and Roberts, D. (1972). *J. Obstet. Gynaec. Br. Commonw.*, **79**, 782.

Crellin, E., Pringle, M. K. and West, P. R. (1971). *Born Illegitimate*, National Foundation for Educational Research, Windsor.

Darwin, C. (1877). *Mind*, **2**, 285.

Davie, R., Butler, N. R. and Goldstein, H. (1972). *From Birth to Seven*, Longman, London.

Dicke, W. K., Weijers, H. A. and van de Kamer, J. H. (1953). *Acta paediat., Stockh.*, **42**, 34.

Douglas, J. W. B. and Blomfield, J. M. (1958). *Children under Five*, Allen & Unwin, London.

Fedrick, J., Alberman, E. and Goldstein, H. (1971). *Nature, Lond.*, **231**, 529.

Goldstein, H. (1973). Personal communication.

Liharzik, F. (1858). *Das Gesetz des menschlichen Wachstumes*, Gerold, Vienna.

Lind, J. (1753). *A Treatise of the Scurvy*, reprinted by Edinburgh University Press, 1953.

Murchison, L. and Larger, S. (1927). *J. Genet. Psychol.*, **34**, 205.

Ounsted, M. and Ounsted, C. (1973). *Clinics, in Developmental Medicine*, No. 46. Heinemann, London.

Rantakallio, P. (1969). *Acta paediat., Stockh.*, **Supp. 193**.

Scammon, R. E. (1927). *Am. J. Physiol. and Anthropology*, **10**, 329.

Simpson, W. J. (1957). *Am. J. Obstet. Gynec.*, **73**, 808.

Spence, J. C., Walton, W. S., Miller, F. J. W. and Court, S. D. M. (1954). *A Thousand Families in Newcastle upon Tyne*, Oxford University Press, Oxford.

Tanner, J. M. (1962). *Growth at Adolescence*, 2nd ed. Blackwell, Oxford.

Yerushalmy, J. (1964). *Am. J. Obstet. Gynec.*, **88**, 505.

Yerushalmy, J. (1971). *Am. J. Epidemiology*, **93**, 443.

Zachau-Christiansen, B. and Ross, E. M. *Development in the First Year of Life*, John Wiley and Sons, Chichester (in press).

CHAPTER 14

Physical factors and mental development

H. GOLDSTEIN

National Children's Bureau, London

INTRODUCTION

The National Child Development Study (NCDS) is a longitudinal survey of the 17 000 children born during 3–9 March 1958 in England, Scotland and Wales. A full description and detailed analyses of the material collected on the children at birth and at seven years can be found in Davie *et al.* (1972). The paper given by Dr Ross today also includes a description of the data collected when the children were 11 years old, in their last year of primary schooling.

Like nearly all large scale surveys the relatively crude nature of the data collected imposes particular constraints upon the analyses which can be carried out. There are, for example, no direct measurements of nutrition, so that it is only possible to make indirect inferences about nutritional influences on, say, mental development, by using surrogates such as height and weight.

However, there is certainly evidence that, for example, height and weight are useful as indirect measurements of nutritional status, even though they are also influenced by other environmental and by genetic factors. The role of such factors will be discussed when the results of the analyses are described below.

HEIGHT, WEIGHT AND ADIPOSITY

Some attention has been given to the problem of finding an index of height and weight which is closely related to adiposity, and therefore to an important aspect of nutritional status (Benn, 1971; Newens and Goldstein 1972). Professor Butler has discussed one such index, namely relative weight, and the factors which are related to it. However, when the relationship of height and weight jointly to mental development is being studied, it does not necessarily follow that the function of height and weight which best predicts adiposity is the same function which best predicts mental development.

The analysis presented here therefore has not used any of the usual weight for height indices such as Quetelet's index or the relative weight. It treats height and weight as separate factors and examines the combination of these which is most closely related to mental development, rather than making the assumption that the relationship can be summarised adequately by using a single index.

FACTORS STUDIED

Apart from any influences on each other, both mental and physical development are influenced separately by additional factors such as social class and birth order. Before attempting, therefore, to speculate on the biological meaning of any relationships it is necessary to understand the role of such intervening or 'nuisance' factors. One way of doing this is to make appropriate statistical allowances, in the present case by analysing the relationship between physical and mental status for fixed sets of values of the 'nuisance' factors. The factors chosen are the social class of the child's father, the numbers of both younger and older children in the child's household, the heights of the parents, the educational level of the parents, and the child's birthweight. A description of the categories of these factors is given in Appendix Table 4.

So far, definitions and measurements of mental development have been avoided. The NCDS used group tests of general ability, reading comprehension and mathematics on the 11 year olds and it is these scores which are used in the following analyses. This paper is not an appropriate place in which to discuss the limitations of such tests, and in particular their cultural biases. We shall assume that, for all their imperfections, differences in average scores between categories of children are useful in indicating differences in the development of reading and mathematics skills and in the overall mental ability summarised in the general ability test.

RESULTS

Figures 1 and 2 show the relationships between mean general ability score and height and weight for boys. Very similar relationships exist for girls and for reading and mathematics test scores. It is clear that the general ability score increases with increasing weight up to about 40 kg with no further increase after that point. For height however there is an increasing relationship over the whole range. In the following analyses, therefore, the height relationship is summarised by a straight line and weight is split into four roughly homogeneous categories as shown in Appendix Table 1.

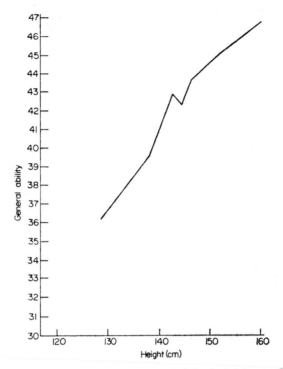

Fig. 1. *Boys,* 11 *years, general ability by height.*

In the first series of analyses, height and weight were analysed jointly, with the three test scores in turn chosen as the 'dependent' variable in an analysis of covariance. These analyses are summarised in Appendix Tables 1–3 and in Figs. 3–5.

It is evident that all three analyses present a similar picture. When allowance is made for height, *i.e.* for fixed values of height, the effect of weight is small, with the highest test scores in the central part of the weight distribution. The gain in test score (in terms of years) per cm increase in height is about the same for all three test scores (5–7 months gain for 10 cm of height), and does not vary with the weight of the child.

The next series of analyses examine whether these relationships can be 'explained' by introducing other related factors. It is known, for example, that working class children, in part for cultural reasons, tend to have lower measured abilities than middle class children. There is also evidence that middle class families tend to provide a better nutritional (growth promoting) environment than working class families. Thus, it is possible that these separate relationships may explain all or part of the observed relationship

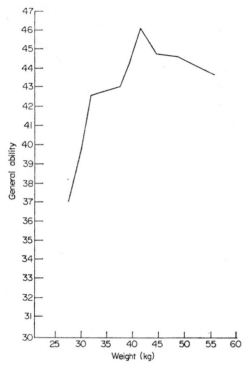

Fig. 2. Boys 11 years, general ability by weight.

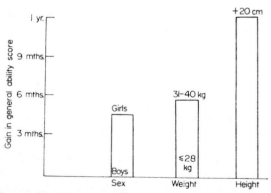

Fig. 3. Height, weight and general ability. Analysis of variance. Differences between extreme groups, i.e. the pair with largest mean difference in score. (N.B. The length of the 'bar' for height is based on a 20 cm difference, which is approximately a range about the mean which includes 80% of the population. This roughly corresponds to the proportion in the central two weight categories.)

between test scores and height and weight. The same reasoning applies to the other factors listed above, and the following analyses examine the extent to which these factors jointly explain the relationships found in the first series of analyses. The results are presented in Figs. 6–8 and Appendix Tables 4–6.

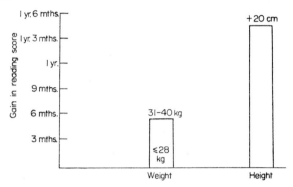

Fig. 4. Height, weight and reading. Analysis of variance. Differences between extreme groups. (See Fig. 3 for explanation.)

Figure 6 shows the combined effect of the factors (where statistically significant) on general ability score. By comparison with Fig. 3 it can be seen that once allowance has been made for all the other factors, the effect of height is reduced by more than one half. The differences between the weight categories are only slightly reduced however. All the other factors studied are statistically significant, except for the parental heights (which on their own are statistically significant but became non-significant when the

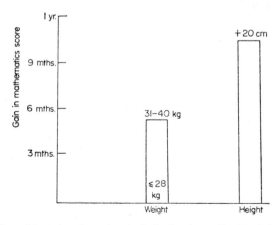

Fig. 5. Height, weight and mathematics. Analysis of variance. (See Fig. 3 for explanation.)

child's weight is allowed for) and, by comparison with both height and weight, the other factors have larger effects on general ability. This can be illustrated by considering a child with a 'disadvantageous' combination of factors, say with four or more younger and four or more older children in the same household, whose father is an unskilled manual worker, and

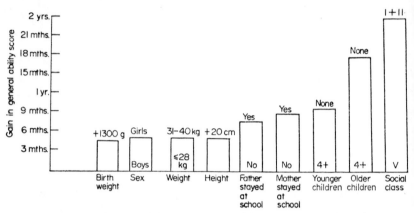

Fig. 6.   Height, weight, general ability and associated factors. (See Fig. 3 for explanation—
birthweight difference also includes approx. 80% of population.)

neither of whose parents stayed on at school after the minimum leaving age. Such a child, is on average over six years behind when compared to a child living with no younger or older children, whose father is in social class I or II and both of whose parents stayed at school after the minimum leaving age. Of course, the proportion of children involved in this comparison is small, but it places the effects of height and weight into perspective.

The effects of height and weight, however, although small, do persist. There appears to be an optimum weight, between 31 and 40 kg where the

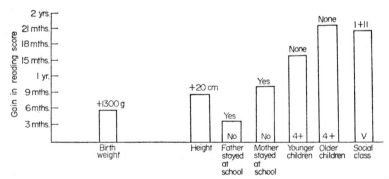

Fig. 7.   Height, weight, reading and associated factors. (See Figs. 3 and 6 for explanation.)

general ability score is highest. The lowest scores, as can be seen also from Fig. 2, are for the light and the heavy children. For height, the general ability score increases with increasing height.

Similar results are found with the reading score (Fig. 7, Appendix Table 5). In this case, the weight effect becomes so small (just over three months of reading) that it is no longer statistically significant. The height coefficient is reduced by half and the average difference between children with 'disadvantageous' and 'advantageous' circumstances is again over six years.

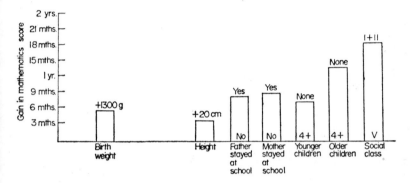

Fig. 8. Height, weight, mathematics and associated factors. (See Figs. 3 and 6 for explanation.)

For arithmetic too there are similar results (Fig. 8, Appendix Table 6). The height coefficient is reduced by over half and the weight effect becomes small and non-significant. The difference between children from 'disadvantageous' and 'advantageous' circumstances is nearly five years.

DISCUSSION

Other research (*see* Tanner, 1963; Scottish Council for Research in Education, 1953) has shown relationships between height and attainment scores with correlation coefficients of about 0·2 as in the present data. Unlike nearly all the previous research, the present paper has considered a number of socio-environmental and biological factors which are related to both height and attainment. In combination these do account for most of the observed association with height, and for reading and arithmetic the relationship with weight becomes negligible. The residual relationship with height might possibly be explained by another factor or set of factors which have not been considered, or it could be a persistent, more fundamental biological relationship which, for example, might be determined in early infancy by the same nutritional factors. A particular nutritional regime might, for example, at the same time affect both physical and mental development, and these effects might persist into later life. Although birthweight, which may be regarded as a crude measure of intrauterine nutrition, is included in the analysis, this has little effect on the observed relationships.

There is also the question of relative maturity factors. It is known (Tanner, 1963) that, especially during puberty, physical growth is related to the degree of physical maturity, which is also related to mental abilities. The children in the NCDS have ratings of pubic hair stages in both boys and girls and breast stages in girls. The relationship of these stages with height and weight is a clear one, as Professor Butler has shown. A further analysis is now in progress to see to what extent the relationship between height and attainment can be accounted for by differences in physical maturity.

SUMMARY AND ABSTRACT

Previous studies have suggested that there may be a 'causal' relationship between measurements of physical status and mental ability. One of the problems is to rule out mutually related factors which may be influencing both measurements but for different reasons. Social class, for example, may be such a factor. It can be argued that working class children have lower measured abilities than middle class children because of cultural differences. It will also be readily accepted that, quite separately, middle class families tend to provide a better nutritional (growth promoting) environment than working class families. In addition it can be argued that both prenatally and in infancy the relative nutritional poverty of working class children contributes both to a lower physical and lower mental status, and is therefore, at least in part, a 'cause' of the relationship.

Measurements of general ability, reading and arithmetic are related to height, weight and a number of social and biological factors, using data on 11-year-old children in the National Child Development Study. It is shown that both height and weight are separately and similarly related to these mental measurements. When allowance is made for the other factors, these relationships are much reduced in size.

REFERENCES

Benn, R. T. (1971). *Br. J. prev. soc. Med.*, **25**, 42.
Davie, R., Butler, N. R., Goldstein, H. (1972). *From Birth to Seven*, Longman, London.
Newens, E. M. and Goldstein, H. (1972). 'Height, weight and the assessment of obesity in children'. *Br. J. prev. soc. Med.*, **26**, 33.

Scottish Council for Research in Education (1953). *Social Implications of the 1947 Scottish Mental Survey*, University of London Press, London.

Tanner, J. M. (1963). *Education and Physical Growth*, University of London Press, London.

APPENDIX

TABLE 1

ANALYSIS OF HEIGHT, WEIGHT AND GENERAL ABILITY SCORE

Dependent variable is general ability score (out of a total score of 80)
Independent variables are:
1. Sex.
2. Height. Continuous variable in centimetres.
3. Weight. 4 categories: 15–28 kg, –31 kg, –40 kg, >40 kg.
Sample size = 5935
Mean score = 43·6

Fitted constants and analysis of variance table
Chi-squared values are adjusted for the other factors

Source	Fitted constant	Standard error	DF	χ^2
Overall constant	52·5			
Sex: boys minus girls	−2·4	0·4	1	34·4[a]
Height coefficient				
(measured about mean = 144·3)	0·32	0·04	1	78·1[a]
Weight: 15–28 kg	−1·7			
–31 kg	0·0			
–40 kg	1·3		3	14·7[b]
>40 kg	0·4			

Test height × weight interaction: $\chi^2 = 3\cdot1$, DF = 3
Residual mean square = 244·0
Total variance   = 252·7

Significance levels
[a] $P < 0\cdot001$
[b] $0\cdot001 < P < 0\cdot01$
[c] $0\cdot01 < P < 0\cdot05$
    otherwise $0\cdot05 < P$

Note: Since the number of degrees of freedom for 'error' are large χ^2 for convenience rather than F values are used. Before carrying out these analyses, the distributions of the test scores were carefully studied to see whether any transformations should be made in order to satisfy statistical assumptions. This discussion will appear in another, more technical, paper, but the overall conclusion was that no transformations were necessary.

TABLE 2

ANALYSIS OF HEIGHT, WEIGHT AND READING COMPREHENSION SCORE

Dependent variable is reading comprehension score (out of a total of 35)
Independent variables are as for Table 1
Sample size = 5935
Mean score = 16·3

Fitted constants and analysis of variance table

Chi-squared values are adjusted for the other factors

Source	Fitted constant	Standard error	DF	χ^2
Overall constant	16·0			
Sex: boys minus girls	0·0	0·1	1	0·0
Height coefficient (measured about mean = 144·3)	0·15	0·01	1	113·7[a]
Weight: 15–28 kg	−0·6			
–31 kg	0·0			
–40 kg	0·4		3	10·9[c]
>40 kg	0·2			

Test height × weight interaction: $\chi^2 = 4\cdot0$, DF = 3
Residual mean square = 37·2
Total variance   = 38·8

TABLE 3

ANALYSIS OF HEIGHT, WEIGHT AND MATHEMATICS SCORE

Dependent variable is mathematics score (out of a total of 40)
Independent variables are as for Table 1
Sample size = 5933
Mean score = 17·1

Fitted constants and analysis of variance table
Chi-squared values are adjusted for the other factors

Source	Fitted constant	Standard error	DF	χ^2
Overall constant	16·4			
Sex: boys minus girls	0·4	0·3	1	1·8
Height coefficient (measured about mean = 144·3)	0·19	0·02	1	65·2[a]
Weight: 15–28 kg	−1·1			
–31 kg	0·0			
–40 kg	0·7		3	9·8[c]
>40 kg	0·4			

Test height $\times$ weight interaction: $\chi^2 = 5·0$, DF = 3
Residual mean square = 103·7
Total variance   = 106·4

TABLE 4

ANALYSIS OF HEIGHT, WEIGHT, ASSOCIATED FACTORS AND GENERAL
ABILITY SCORE

Dependent variable is general ability score
Independent variables are:

1. Sex.
2. Height. Continuous variable in centimetres.
3. Weight. 4 categories: 15–28 kg, –31 kg, –40 kg, >40 kg.
4. Social class. 5 categories (Registrar General, 1960):
     I + II, III non-manual, III manual, IV, V.
5. Number of older children in child's household. 4 categories: 0, 1, 2–3, 4+.
6. Number of younger children in child's household. 4 categories: 0, 1, 2–3, 4+.
7. Mother's height. Continuous variable in centimetres (measured at birth).
8. Father's height. Continuous variable in centimetres (enquired at 11).
9. Whether mother stayed on at school after minimum school leaving age.
     2 categories: yes, no.
10. Whether father stayed on at school after minimum school leaving age.
     2 categories: yes, no.
11. Birthweight. Continuous variable in grammes.

Sample size = 4333
Mean score = 44·3

Fitted constants and analysis of variance table
Chi-squared values are adjusted for the other factors

Source	Fitted constant	Standard error	DF	χ^2
Overall constant	35·5			
Sex: boys minus girls	−2·6	0·4	1	34·2[a]
Height coefficient (measured about mean = 144·3)	0·12	0·04	1	8·5[b]
Weight: 15–28 kg	−1·3			
−31 kg	0·3		3	15·4[b]
−40 kg	1·3			
>40 kg	−0·3			
Social class: I + II	4·7			
III nm	3·0			
III m	1·9		4	122·0[a]
IV	−1·8			
V	−7·8			
Older children: 0	4·2			
1	1·6		3	98·9[a]
2–3	−0·9			
4+	−4·9			

continued

Younger children: 0	2·3			
1	1·2		3	38·1[a]
2–3	−0·5			
4+	−3·0			
Mother's height coefficient (measured about mean = 162·0 cm)	0·11	0·48	1	0·1
Father's height coefficient (measured about mean = 174·6 cm)	0·19	0·40	1	0·2
Mother stayed at school: yes minus no	4·8	0·5	1	77·2[a]
Father stayed at school: yes minus no	4·1	0·6	1	46·2[a]
Birthweight coefficient (measured about mean = 3395 g)	0·0018	0·0004	1	15·3[a]

Test height $\times$ weight interaction: $\chi^2 = 5\cdot0$, DF $= 3$
Residual mean square $= 204\cdot0$
Total variance $= 246\cdot2$
Fitting all variables except weight:
height coefficient $= 0\cdot12$, standard error $= 0\cdot03$, $\chi^2 = 13\cdot4^a$
Fitting mother's height alone:
coefficient $= 2\cdot4$, standard error $= 0\cdot5$, $\chi^2 = 22\cdot0^a$
Fitting father's height alone:
coefficient $= 2\cdot7$, standard error $= 0\cdot4$, $\chi^2 = 42\cdot0^a$

Note: Since the average test scores change with age it is useful to present contrasts between the levels of the independent variables in terms of the equivalent number of years. Data are available, from the tests used, of the average increase per year at round 11 years of age, and are as follows:

general ability	6·3 points per year
reading	2·2 points per year
mathematics	4·5 points per year

These estimates are used in the construction of Figs. 3–8.

TABLE 5

ANALYSIS OF HEIGHT, WEIGHT, ASSOCIATED FACTORS AND READING SCORE

Dependent variable is reading comprehension score
Independent variables are as for Table 4
Sample size = 4333
Mean score = 16·5

Fitted constant and analysis of variance table
Chi-squared values are adjusted for the other factors

Source	Fitted constant	Standard error	DF	χ^2
Overall constant	13·0			
Sex: boys minus girls	0·2	0·2	1	0·9
Height coefficient (measured about mean = 144·3)	0·08	0·02	1	24·9[a]
Weight: 15–28 kg	−0·3			
–31 kg	0·1			
–40 kg	0·3		3	7·3
>40 kg	−0·1			
Social class: I + II	1·8			
III nm	1·4			
III m	−0·2			
IV	−0·9		4	135·6[a]
V	−2·1			

continued

Older children: 0	2·0			
1	0·4			
2–3	−0·3		3	153·5[a]
4+	−2·1			
Younger children: 0	1·4			
1	0·4			
2–3	−0·3		3	85·6[a]
4+	−1·5			
Mother's height coefficient (measured about mean = 162·0 cm)	−0·10	0·19	1	0·3
Father's height coefficient (measured about mean = 174·6 cm)	0·04	0·16	1	0·1
Mother stayed at school: yes minus no	2·0	0·2	1	92·9[a]
Father stayed at school: yes minus no	0·8	0·2	1	44·4[a]
Birthweight coefficient (measured about mean = 3395 g)	0·0008	0·0002	1	21·3[a]

Test height $\times$ weight interaction: $\chi^2 = 7\cdot0$, DF $= 3$
Residual mean square $= 30\cdot3$
Total variance $\quad\quad = 38\cdot1$
Fitting all variables except weight:
height coefficient $= 0\cdot08$, standard error $= 0\cdot01$, $\chi^2 = 35\cdot5^a$
Fitting mother's height alone:
coefficient $= 1\cdot0$, standard error $= 0\cdot2$, $\chi^2 = 23\cdot4^a$
Fitting father's height alone:
coefficient $= 1\cdot2$, standard error $= 0\cdot2$, $\chi^2 = 49\cdot6^a$

TABLE 6

ANALYSIS OF HEIGHT, WEIGHT, ASSOCIATED FACTORS AND MATHEMATICS
SCORE

Dependent variable is mathematics score
Independent variables are as for Table 4
Sample size = 4331
Mean score = 17·5

Fitted constant and analysis of variance table
Chi-squared values are adjusted for the other factors

Source	Fitted constant	Standard error	DF	χ^2
Overall constant	12·4			
Sex: boys minus girls	0·15	0·29	1	0·3
Height coefficient (measured about mean = 144·3)	0·07	0·03	1	5·9[c]
Weight: 15–28 kg	−0·5			
−31 kg	0·1			
−40 kg	0·5		3	4·8
>40 kg	−0·1			
Social class: I + II	3·2			
III nm	2·3			
III m	−0·1		4	146·4[a]
IV	−1·6			
V	−3·8			

continued

Older children: 0	2·3			
1	0·8			
2–3	−0·4		3	71·1[a]
4+	−2·7			
Younger children: 0	1·3			
1	0·4			
2–3	−0·4		3	26·4[a]
4+	−1·3			
Mother's height coefficient (measured about mean = 162·0 cm)	0·1	0·3	1	0·1
Father's height coefficient (measured about mean = 174·6 cm)	−0·3	0·3	1	1·4
Mother stayed at school: yes minus no	3·5	0·4	1	100·9[a]
Father stayed at school: yes minus no	3·0	0·4	1	59·1[a]
Birthweight coefficient (measured about mean = 3395 g)	0·0015	0·0003	1	28·0[a]

Test height $\times$ weight interaction: $\chi^2 = 6·5$, DF $= 3$
Residual mean square $= 85·8$
Total variance $\qquad = 104·7$
Fitting all variables except weight:
height coefficient $= 0·07$, standard error $= 0·02$, $\chi^2 = 9·9$[a]
Fitting mother's height alone:
coefficient $= 1·6$, standard error $= 0·3$, $\chi^2 = 23·4$[a]
Fitting father's height alone:
coefficient $= 1·4$, standard error $= 0·3$, $\chi^2 = 27·0$[a]

PART 4

FOOD FOR ADULTS:

HOW MUCH AND OF WHAT KIND?
IS THERE A CASE FOR FORTIFICATION?

CHAPTER 15

Energy foods

D. S. PARSONS

Department of Biochemistry, University of Oxford

INTRODUCTION

Energy foods represent the inputs to complex multistep systems of energy homeostasis in living animals. The energy foods consumed are not necessarily the immediate fuels of combustion which provide the power required to drive fundamental cellular processes. The energy currency in cells is the terminal pyrophosphate bond in ATP. Energy foods are combusted in order to provide this cellular energy currency, and about 84 kJ (20 kcal) of energy food are required per mole of $\sim P$ yield. Frequently an input of energy occurs in one chemical form which is then subjected to further transformations before combustion so that energy foods may be broken down and reassembled in a different way for storage. It follows from these considerations that it is impossible to discuss energy foods without consideration of the total picture of energy homeostasis.

NATURE OF ENERGY REQUIREMENTS

The overall energy requirements of animals may be divided into two, namely basal requirements and work requirements. The basal requirements are those necessary to sustain the organisation and operation of the metabolic systems (*e.g.* ion pumping, membrane synthesis, protein synthesis) of the animal. Work requirements are those imposed by work loads undertaken by the animal in achieving tasks during interactions with the environment. It appears that ion pumping processes can account for more than 50% of the basal requirements (Whittam, 1964; Milligan, 1971). The energy necessary to sustain the turnover of the tissue proteins accounts for 15% of basal requirements (Milligan, 1971). Related to the overall requirements are the consequences of the efficiency of the utilisation of energy by animals, for example the ratio (power output/power input) for the basal and for work requirements (the machine efficiency). The machine efficiency of ionic pumping appears to be about 60% (Milligan, 1971), while for muscle it is 25–35% (Kushmerick and Davies, 1969; Kushmerick *et al.*, 1969). The efficiency of energy storage and of the mobilisation of these stores, an obligatory consequence of the fact that energy input and output do not usually coincide in time, has also to be considered. The yield of high energy phosphate in the form of ATP from different sources is given in Table 1.

TABLE 1

YIELD OF HIGH ENERGY PHOSPHATE AS ATP FROM DIFFERENT SOURCES

Substrate	Moles of high energy phosphate ($\sim P$) per mole of substrate metabolised
Glucose	36
Propionate	18
Butyrate	27
Stearic acid	146
100 g protein	23

ENERGY HOMEOSTASIS

A fundamental, but trivial, thermodynamic statement is that

$$\text{energy input} = \text{energy output} + \text{energy stored}$$

The fact is that over a period of time most adult humans maintain a steady state of energy balance with a constant quantity of energy stored. In other words the rate of energy input in the form of energy foods very nearly equals the rate of output of energy over a period of time. The maintenance of this homeostasis is such that, for example over a 365 day period, a 1% error in the intake of energy foods will induce a change in bodyweight of about 2 kg (as adipose tissue) and a 0·1% error in homeostasis would represent a change in bodyweight of about 200 g (Table 2).

TABLE 2

ENERGY HOMEOSTASIS

With an intake of energy foods equivalent to 12·6 MJ (3000 kcal) per day, over a year this will amount to 4600 MJ ($1·1 \times 10^6$ kcal). If energy homeostasis is in error by 1%, less being expended than consumed, then 46 MJ ($1·1 \times 10^4$ kcal) will be stored as lipid. 46 MJ is the energetic value of approximately 1 kg of triglyceride and will be contained in about 2 kg of adipose tissue.

SPECIES VARIATION IN RATE OF CONSUMPTION OF ENERGY FOODS

	Bodyweight (kg)	Period of food intake (min/day)	Per cent of day spent consuming food	Energy consumption (MJ (kcal)/24 hours)	Rate of input of energy (kJ (kcal)/kg bodyweight/min)
Carnivores					
Lion	250	17	1·1	38·6 (9 213)	9·2 (2·2)
Leopard	75	12	0·9	12·9 (3 071)	14·2 (3·4)
Fox	5·5	8	0·5	1·7 (413)	39·8 (9·5)
Omnivores					
Boar	200	40	2·8	20·3 (4 843)	2·6 (0·61)
Badger	9	31	2·1	5·4 (1 299)	19·7 (4·7)
Herbivores					
Zebra	340	405	28·1	14·6 (3 491)	0·13 (0·03)
Pony	125	414	28·9	15·2 (3 642)	0·29 (0·07)
Sheep	70	155	13·0	6·6 (1 573)	0·63 (0·14)
Hare	5	234	16·2	1·3 (317)	1·1 (0·26)
Human					
Oxford don resident in college	80	110	7·6	12·1 (2 900)	1·4 (0·33)
Male graduate student:					
weekday	70	40	2·7	10·5 (2 500)	3·7 (0·89)
Sunday		80	5·6	11·3 (2 700)	2·0 (0·48)

Includes data of Fábry (1969). A leopard, when eating, consumes energy foods at 10 times the rate of an Oxford don, who in turn consumes kilojoules at about twice the rate of a sheep.

ENERGY INPUT—EPISODIC

The input of energy to animals is discontinuous, *i.e.* periodic; in complete contrast, energy expenditure is continuous, being composed of basal expenditure with added episodes of additional expenditure related to external work. In some cases the capture of energy foods requires considerable energy expenditure. Thus in hunting there may be a positive feedback relating expenditure and intake. In highly organised societies the acquisition of energy foods seems to require minimum expenditure of energy.

The duration of time over which the energy input to the body occurs varies remarkably among different species, and in human subjects, within different races and social and occupational groups. Generally speaking, carnivorous animals expend a very small fraction of their life assimilating energy; this may amount to less than 1% of life (Table 3). In contrast, herbivorous animals may spend up to 20% of their life eating. Time spent in the acquisition of energy by human subjects is extremely variable, depending on factors such as occupation, social status, age, income and disposition; the average adult appears to spend something like 5% of life eating. Between different subjects, however, there seems to be much variation in how this time is allocated during the day.

It is possible to divide human subjects into two types, the 'nibblers' and the 'stuffers'. Nibblers are persons who take a number of relatively small meals—we may perhaps call them snacks—each day, for example up to six or seven throughout the day. The stuffers are at the other extreme, and they eat one large or very large meal once a day or even less frequently.

TABLE 4

INFLUENCE OF MEAL FREQUENCY ON ENERGY INTAKE AND PHYSIQUE. DATA CALCULATED FROM FABRY (1969), ARE OF MEANS ±SEM. TOTAL NUMBER OF SUBJECTS, 89

Average frequency of meals/24 hours	Energy intake/day (MJ (kcal))	Bodyweight (kg)	Abdominal skinfold thickness (cm)
3–4	15·0 ± 0·3 (3 580)	83 ± 1	2·6 ± 0·1
4–5	16·6 ± 0·3 (3 960)	80 ± 1	2·3 ± 0·1
5–6	18·3 ± 0·1 (4 381)	77 ± 1	2·0 ± 0·1

Fábry (1969) has examined this aspect of eating behaviour and, not surprisingly, he finds a positive correlation between the number of meals a day and energy input. Interestingly, however, there is a negative correlation between the number of meals a day and bodyweight and also with the skinfold thickness (Table 4). There is also a negative correlation between the number of meals a day and the plasma cholesterol level and the incidence of ischaemic heart disease (Fábry, 1969). It seems to me that much more work requires to be done on this aspect of nutrition in an attempt to discover whether the jobs undertaken by nibblers are such that they are forced to take frequent small meals or whether the food intake follows some constitutional makeup and is associated with a propensity to low bodyweight and so forth. It would be interesting to compare the extent and duration of output of the gastrointestinal hormones in the two groups of subjects. There are also other questions which seem to me to be capable of investigation in humans. For example: if the first meal of the day is large, are people hungrier and do they eat more during the rest of the day? Also, with supplies of energy foods not rate limiting, is the individual intake at a communal meal greater than when the meal is taken alone? (The 'pig trough' effect.)

ENERGY EXPENDITURE—CONTINUOUS

Because the utilisation of energy is a continuing requirement to which are added episodes of augmentation, animals must contain systems for storing and transporting energy. Closely associated, therefore, with the concept of energy foods is the problem of the nature of the energy stores and the nature of the forms in which energy foods are transported between intestine, the energy stores and the tissues. Two factors determine the daily

TABLE 5

EFFECTS OF SLEEP DURATION ON TOTAL ENERGY EXPENDITURE

Sleeping (hours/day)	Total energy expenditure (MJ/24 hours)		
	Sedentary	Moderately active	Very active
3	10·5	16·3	20·7
4	10·4	15·8	20·0
5	10·2	15·4	19·4
6	10·0	15·0	18·7
7	9·9	14·5	18·1
8	9·7	14·0	17·4
9	9·5	13·6	16·8
10	9·4	13·2	16·1

Assumptions:

Rate of metabolism while awake—kJ (kcal)/hour
    sedentary: 460 (110)
    moderately active: 753 (175)
    very active: 942 (225)
Rate of metabolism during sleep—293 kJ (70 kcal)/hour

expenditure of energy. One factor is the nature of the work done on the environment by the individual, which in turn is related to the ethnic group, the place in society and method of food acquisition. The other factor is the amount of sleep taken by the individual.

Duration of sleep varies considerably with different individuals, and this must have an influence on the overall utilisation of energy. The effects of duration of sleep on energy utilisation will vary, depending on whether the subjects involved are 'stuffers' or 'nibblers'. Presumably nibblers will automatically reduce their intake of energy because the extent of eating in such subjects could be directly proportional to the hours of wakefulness, but not so the stuffers (Table 5). Here again is a field where more experimentation is required.

It is of interest in this connection that there may be some relationship between gastrointestinal hormone output and sleep. Postprandial sleepiness may thus have an endocrinological basis (Fara *et al.*, 1969; Březinová and Oswald, 1972; Southwell *et al.*, 1972).

ENERGY STORAGE

Implied in the concept of an episodic input of energy in subjects continuously expending energy is the fact that energy is stored and transported, so that the path of energy transformation involves the following steps

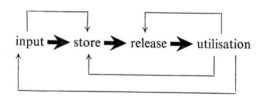

Feedbacks evidently operate on this path, and again much is yet to be learned about how these operate. There seems to be some relationship between energy utilisation and input (*see* section on energy input) and the gastrointestinal hormones themselves may switch on storage and switch off release processes (Creutzfeldt, 1970).

NATURE OF ENERGY INPUTS AND THEIR TRANSFORMATIONS

Fats and carbohydrates are the major energy foods. However, because of the interconversion of amino acids to glucose, proteins themselves must be included as energy foods; the protein-sparing effects of carbohydrates have long been known.

In discussing transport and storage of energy foods three stages can be defined. These are the absorptive stage, the postabsorptive stage and starvation.

Lipids are absorbed into the intestinal mucosa as mono- and diglycerides and transported in the lymph, mainly as chylomicra. These consist of triglyceride oil droplets with an amphipathic surround composed of phospholipids and proteins, and are synthesised in the intestinal mucosal cells (Johnston, 1968). The fact that triglyceride enters the body via the lymphatic system means that the fat does not go directly to the liver but bypasses it. In the capillary beds of the peripheral tissues, especially adipose tissue, the triglyceride is hydrolysed to free fatty acids and glycerol. Free fatty acids easily enter tissues, and can be oxidised or, in adipose tissue, re-esterified.

Carbohydrate is absorbed into the intestinal mucosal cells, chiefly as disaccharide, *i.e.* as maltose, sucrose and lactose. There are large racial differences between the nature of carbohydrate energy foods that are ingested. For example, in many parts of the world lactose is absent from the diet, and intestinal lactase deficiency is well recognised in these areas. Civilisation, sophistication and sucrose intake appear to go together, and recently there has been much discussion as to whether continuing high levels of sucrose intake have deleterious effects.

In the case of carbohydrate, energy-yielding substrate is transported in the blood as the monosaccharide glucose. Glucose is stored in the liver in its polymeric form, glycogen, from which it can be released as glucose again, or in muscle also as glucagon, but from which the carbohydrate is released into blood only as lactate. The energy available in carbohydrate can also be stored in adipose tissue after conversion to free fatty acids and subsequent esterification.

During the absorptive state the energy stores are, as it were, topped up, and in the postabsorptive state these energy stores are full and ready for release during starvation. Insulin appears to be the principal storage hormone, but gastrointestinal hormones may have important controlling influences on storage. The gastrointestinal hormones certainly can augment the release of insulin, even before the blood sugar starts to rise (Creutzfeldt, 1970). Insulin acts to promote the uptake and storage of fat in adipose tissues. This follows because insulin inhibits the mobilisation of adipose tissue fatty acids, as a result of a specific inhibition of the adipose tissue lipase. As a result, the utilisation of glucose by peripheral tissues is facilitated, and the utilisation of fatty acids inhibited in the stage when storage is occurring. Thus, during absorption and in the immediate postabsorptive state, carbohydrate is a primary metabolic fuel. In the late postabsorptive state, and in starvation, energy stores are mobilised in the form of free fatty acids, and because fatty acids inhibit glucose utilisation the energy fuels change from carbohydrate to fat; and in the liver most of the free fatty acids are converted to ketone bodies. Also, following the mobilisation of amino acids from tissues, and of glycerol from adipose tissues, gluconeogenesis occurring in the liver and kidney is the source of the blood sugar. In starvation, therefore, the primary metabolic fuels of most tissues are fatty acids and the ketone bodies. However, certain tissues require for their correct functioning a continuous supply of glucose. These are, notably, the central nervous system, erythrocytes, and perhaps the intestinal mucosa. During starvation the ketones are increasingly utilised, and because of the high levels of mobilised fat in the blood there may be a greater input of energy in the form of fat and ketone bodies into the muscles than they need. The result is that fat may actually become deposited in the muscles.

TABLE 6

ENERGETIC EFFICIENCY OF STORAGE

(Data of Milligan, 1971)

Precursors Substrate (moles)	$\sim P$ (moles)	Product (moles)	Cost of storage %[a]
Average amino acid (1)	4	Protein (100 g)	11
Glucose (1) + glycogen (n − 1)	2	Glycogen (n)	3
Glucose (2)	2	Lactose (1)	2
Glucose (12·5)	34	Triglyceride (tripalmitin) (1)	17
Acetate (8)	43	Palmitate (1)	29
Palmitate (3) + glycerol (1)	8	Tripalmitin (1)	3

[a] Calculated as:

$$100 \times \frac{\text{(precursor energy)} - \text{(product energy)}}{\text{precursor energy}}$$

NB: Numbers in parentheses equal the number of moles.

As regards the chemical nature of the energy stores it should be noted that fat is about 40 times more energy-dense than carbohydrate and several times more dense than acetate in isotonic solution. There are no specific protein stores, and muscle and perhaps liver will supply amino acids for gluconeogenesis. It is of interest that the efficiency of conversion of glucose to triglyceride is less than that of the conversion of glucose to glycogen (Table 6). Some estimates of the size of energy stores in humans are given in Table 7.

TABLE 7

ESTIMATES OF APPROXIMATE ENERGY RESERVES IN 65-KG MALE SUBJECTS

(*see also* Passmore, 1969)

Energy reserve in the form of *triglyceride*:
    8 kg = 300 MJ (72 Mcal)
Energy reserve in the form of *carbohydrate*:

Muscle 30 kg, 5 g CHO/kg	150 g
Liver 1·5 kg, 50 g CHO/kg	75 g
Extracellular fluid 15 litres	
1 g CHO/litre	15 g
	240 g

giving a total energy reserve in the form of carbohydrate 3·8 MJ (900 kcal)
Protein as energy reserve:
    With lean cell mass 39 kg, and if one-third of this can be 'utilised' for
    gluconeogenesis the energy 'store' in this form is 13 kg giving an energy
    reserve of 217 MJ (50 Mcal)
With an energy utilisation rate of, say, 10 MJ/day, the reserves will amount to:

Triglyceride	30 days' supply
Carbohydrate <	1 day's supply
Protein	20 days' supply

NOVEL ENERGY FOODS

Lipids are the most energy-dense substances and very expensive; in a world facing an ever-increasing shortage of energy supplies it is worth considering novel energetic foodstuffs.

One such way is for the food industry to search for a means of isolating and preparing on a large scale lipids from algal and other vegetable sources which are both palatable and non-toxic. Another possible way might be the induction of caecal/colonic fermentation in human subjects on a scale sufficiently large to enable cellulose to be utilised at a significant rate. It is a characteristic of caecal fermenters that cellulose is fermented to lower fatty acids such as acetate and butyrate. Indeed, a large fraction of the energy intake of herbivorous animals occurs in this form (Henning and Hird, 1972*a*, *b*). It is well known that ruminants obtain the whole of their energy intake in the form of volatile fatty acids by the absorption of the products of rumen fermentation from the forestomach (Annison and Lewis, 1959).

Although there seems to be a negative correlation between the bulkiness of the diet and colonic disease (Burkitt *et al.*, 1972) the consumption of large quantities of *e.g.* cellulose will lead to the presence in the small intestine of large quantities of unabsorbable polyvalent ions. This may give rise to problems *e.g.* binding of important nutrients. Nevertheless, the possibility of inducing caecal fermentation on a relatively large scale to supply energy in human subjects should be considered.

For a long term solution my view is that the world shortage of energy foodstuffs could be solved by entirely new procedures in which the energy of the sun (*see* Table 8) is directly trapped on a large scale by the use of

TABLE 8

WORLD ENERGY SUPPLIES AND TOTAL HUMAN ENERGY REQUIREMENTS COMPUTED FOR WORLD POPULATION OF 10^9 SOULS. DATA FOR ENERGY SOURCES CALCULATED FROM FOX AND DOSE (1972). ENERGY REQUIREMENTS OF 1 SOUL ASSUMED TO BE 1.05×10^7 J/DAY (2.5×10^6 CAL/DAY)

Energy requirements	J/year
Annual requirements	
1 soul	3.8×10^9
World population of 10^9 souls	3.8×10^{18}

Energy supplies	
Source	
Total optical solar radiation	5.4×10^{24}
Solar radiation below 200 nm	1.6×10^{21}
High energy radiation from earth's crust	3.3×10^{20}
Energy from electrical discharges	8.4×10^{19}
Heat from volcanic emissions	3.1×10^{18}

techniques of applied biochemistry. In other words, I envisage the establishment of giant, self-supporting ecosystems, in which chloroplasts cultured on a vast industrial scale fix CO_2 to produce carbohydrate, which would be harvested and added directly to the diet. Once ecosystems of this sort are established I can really see no reason why further transformations of the carbohydrate, *e.g.* a direct synthesis *in vitro* of triglyceride, should not be feasible propositions.

CONCLUSIONS

The energy requirements of animals are basal requirements plus work requirements. Basal requirements are those for ionic pumping processes and turnover of tissue protein. Energy requirements and energy availability are to some extent linked in a positive feedback servosystem in that work required to capture food increases the energetic requirements. Over the long term, energy input equals the energy expenditure plus the energy stored, and the homeostasis achieved in practice is excellent in human subjects. For a man expending 10·5 MJ (2500 kcal) a day, an error of 0·1 % in regulation will amount to 37·7 MJ (9000 kcal) a year, equivalent to a loss or gain of about 100 g triglyceride; *i.e.* a change of 0·25 kg in bodyweight in the form of adipose tissue.

Energy input on a short term basis is episodic. Food is taken in over a short period and then stored, principally as triglyceride. Time spent in eating depends on the nature of the animal, but in the 70 kg range of bodyweight a carnivore, *e.g.* leopard, spends 1 % of the day eating, whereas a university professor spends 7% and a sheep 13% of the day eating. Entry of food into the gastrointestinal tract may activate early warning systems which switch on storage and switch off mobilisation of energetic foodstuffs. Organic polymers of the diet are broken down by digestion into constituent monomers, which are stored in a dense form. Energy density in adipose tissue is 40 times that of glucose and nearly 300 times that of sodium acetate in isotonic solution. Individual steps of storage are relatively highly efficient, but the overall cost of storage of glucose as triglyceride is about 20% of the energy value. Efficiency of utilisation of metabolic energy for mechanical work is about 30%, but for ion transport it may be more than 50%. The transport of energy between different organs occurs in the bloodstream in two principal forms, as glucose or as free fatty acids and ketones. In the absorptive state, carbohydrate is taken up by most tissues and seems to be the preferred energy food. In later stages, utilisation of glucose is confined to the central nervous system and highly specialised tissues such as erythrocytes, other tissues using as preferred fuel fatty acids and ketones. Novel energy foods are considered, and it is suggested that a possible long-term solution to a world shortage of energy foods may be a form of farming by ecosystems *in vitro*. From such systems carbohydrates and lipids would be harvested as crops of high energy foods derived from the transduction of solar energy through the use of chloroplasts cultured *in vitro*.

REFERENCES

Annison, D. F. and Lewis, D. (1959). *Metabolism in the Rumen*, Methuen, London.

Březinová, V. and Oswald, I. (1972). *Br. med. J.*, **2**, 431.

Burkitt, D. P., Walker, A. R. P. and Painter, N. S. (1972). *Lancet*, **2**, 1408.

Creutzfeldt, W. (1970). Editor *Origin, Chemistry, Physiology and Pathophysiology of the Gastrointestinal Hormones*, Schattauer Verlag, Stuttgart.

Fábry, P. (1969). *Feeding Pattern and Nutritional Adaptations*, Butterworth, London.

Fara, J. W., Rubinstein, E. M. and Sonnenschein, R. R. (1969). *Science*, **166**, 110.

Fox, S. W. and Dose, K. (1972). In: *Molecular Evolution and the Origin of Life*, Ch. 3. W. H. Freeman & Co., San Francisco.

Henning, S. J. and Hird, F. J. R. (1972a). *Biochem. J.*, **130**, 785.

Henning, S. J. and Hird, F. J. R. (1972b). *Biochem. J.*, **130**, 791.

Johnston, J. M. (1968). In *Handbook of Physiology*, edited by C. F. Code, Section 6, Vol. 3, Ch. 70, p. 1313. Am. Physiol. Society, Washington D.C.

Kushmerick, M. J. and Davies, R. E. (1969). *Proc. Roy. Soc. Lond., Ser. B.*, **174**, 315.

Kushmerick, M. J., Larson, R. E. and Davies, R. E. (1969). *Proc. Roy. Soc. Lond., Ser. B.*, **174**, 293.

Milligan, L. P. (1971). *Fed. Proc.*, **30**, 1454.

Passmore, R. (1969). Appendix I in *Recommended Intakes of Nutrients for the United Kingdom*, HMSO, London.

Southwell, P. R., Evans, C. R. and Hunt, J. N. (1972). *Br. med. J.*, **2**, 429.

Whittam, R. (1964). In *The Cellular Functions of Membrane Transport*, edited by J. F. Hoffman, p. 139, Prentice-Hall, Englewood Cliffs, N.J.

CHAPTER 16

Protein foods

A. SPICER

Director of Research, The Lord Rank Research Centre, High Wycombe

It would probably be a mistake to give a paper on 'Protein Foods'—
which I think would be better labelled 'Novel Protein Foods'—within the
framework of a nutrition conference without touching, however briefly,
on the *raison d'être* for such new nutrient sources in a world which appears
in many regions amply supplied with food and, in some regions, even over-
supplied. In meeting after meeting, we refer to pockets—large or small—
of malnutrition in the rich or developed countries, quite apart from inci-
dents of kwashiorkor or marasmus in the poor or underdeveloped nations,
thus indicating that faulty nutrition is not a scientific or economic problem
only but one of food habits, religious beliefs, taboos and many other facets
which are not inherent in illiterate or semi-educated men only but persist
equally in the most advanced society. Though food science and nutrition
have for some decades now established themselves as respectable scientific
disciplines, food *per se*, what to eat and what not to eat, is still approached
by man with a great deal of mysticism and only large scale nutritional
education, stretching over a generation or longer, may bring about a
more rational approach for the benefit of all mankind. Whilst we accept,
therefore, that a multitude of reasons cause nutritional problems of one
kind or another, we cannot be in any doubt about the effect of the population growth on the supply situation of macronutrients.

In a number of reports by FAO and other organisations, the total arable
land available for agriculture is about 3200 million hectares. According to
the type of crop grown, the husbandry applied and the level of consumption,
0·5 to 0·9 hectares per person are required and all arable land will be under
cultivation by the end of the century to feed the 6000 million mouths
then to be fed. Better agronomical conditions will, without doubt, improve
this situation but the margin, even under the most optimistic measurements, does not appear to be a very wide one.

Figure 1 highlights a particular area of concern for us as scientists
working in the field of nutrition, namely protein, since photosynthesis
could and will supply our needs for carbohydrates as the major source
of our energy in a variety of forms in different parts of the world. There
appears for the moment no foreseeable worry regarding the availability of
the third macronutrient, namely lipids, and I would like to show you some

forecasts for this raw material made by the Ministry of Agriculture, Fisheries and Food (Table 1).

Paul Lachance of Rutgers University, New Brunswick, calls this whole rush to discover new protein sources in America a somewhat idiotic and unnecessary scramble based on misinformation about nutritional needs. It

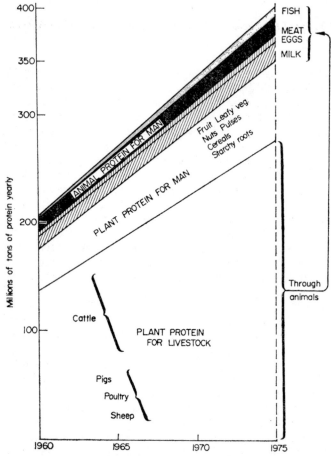

Fig. 1. *World protein production—present and projected.*

is true that millions of Americans eat too much protein; it is true that our estimates for optimal requirements for this nutrient are probably higher than the minimal requirements which would ensure a sound balanced nutrient supply to the average man. We know that hundreds of millions of people have a lower protein intake than appears to be indicated and they appear to have a proper development to maturity. What we cannot assess, in the absence of proper epidemiological studies, is their resistance to disease and their eligibility for an extended and disease free old age which, together with a satisfactory development in youth, would be synonymous with the supply of an adequate diet.

TABLE 1

FEED EQUIVALENTS AVAILABLE IN EXCESS OF MAN'S NEEDS

(metric tons $\times$ 10^6)

	1965	1975	1985	2000
Cereal equivalent	541	541	508	475
Oilseed equivalent	96	103	110	123

Based on 1·7% compound world population increase.

We would therefore have to accept that, owing to varying circumstances, a case for an increasing demand for new protein sources has been established, particularly at a price people can afford to pay. This demand will grow by 10% or more per annum, if these last 12 months are considered a meaningful guideline.

We know today—or at least we appear to know—the quantity and quality of protein man must ingest to survive. We also know that there are quite special requirements for protein quality and quantity:

1. for the expectant mother;
2. for the newly born; and
3. for the growing child.

Extensive clinical research in many parts of the world has also indicated that protein malnutrition of the expectant mother and the newly born may not only have irreversible growth-stunting effects on the neonate, but also persistent effects on measured intelligence and learning basic skills. Survivors of early protein malnutrition are different from normal children.

The quantitative requirements of ordinary adults are 35–50 g or about 1½–2 oz/day and, on the quality side, we now know that we must obtain the essential amino acids from ingested foods since the body cannot synthesise them. These amino acids are essential for tissue building and therefore for the maintenance of body function.

Our endeavour to find new protein sources will, to a fair extent, be based on agriculture and there protein concentrates or isolates from higher plants will without doubt make quantitatively the most important contribution to the protein supply in the human diet for some time to come.

Why concentrates rather than whole plants?

1. The raw material of the whole plant may be unacceptable as human food (leaf or grass).
2. The raw material may contain, together with the protein, toxic substances or too much indigestible raw fibre which has to be removed.
3. Often protein concentrates are formed during the recovery of other valuable food components, such as lipids or starch (oilseeds or gluten separation).
4. With the availability of protein concentrates it becomes possible to compose more reliable foods by the proper combination of food components in order to obtain a better diet.
5. Concentrates can form high protein foods on their own or can be used for upgrading low protein foods.
6. Supplementation with missing amino acids can improve biological values.

Which protein concentrates are we talking about?

LEAF PROTEIN

Pirie's group at Rothamsted and others have made systematic and consistent efforts in developing the techniques of leaf protein production aiming mainly at human consumption. The isolation process consists essentially of the preparation of extracts from fresh vegetation. Fresh plants are pulped with a suitable pulper and this pulp is pressed giving an extract from which the proteins are coagulated by heating. This is followed by separating, washing and pressing the coagulated proteins which have to be preserved. In this way, 50% or more of the total proteins in green plants can be recovered in a 60–70% protein concentrate.

In the process as outlined, the greater part of the soluble nutrients, such as amino acids, sugar, vitamins and minerals are lost in the effluent after the coagulation of the proteins. A flowsheet of a similar production process by Hollo and co-workers is shown in Fig. 2.

GRASS PROTEIN

The same workers developed a multistage pressing process for alfalfa and from the pressed liquor the protein is coagulated by heating to give a curd of 25–30% solids and the whey liquor is vacuum concentrated to 55–70% dry matter. Curd and whey concentrates are then mixed together and spray-dried, retaining as the end product about 70% of the nutritional value of the green plant.

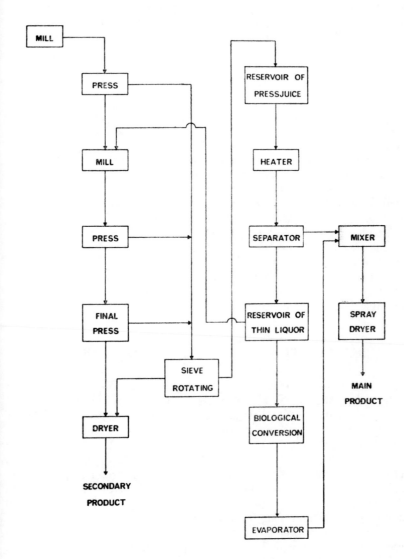

Fig. 2. Flowsheet of leaf protein concentrate process.

Both the leaf and the grass protein hold out a fair promise, yet far more nutritional and biochemical information is needed about these substances before they could really be regarded as safe for human consumption. Their bitter flavour and colour are also strong points against them.

GLUTEN

The next protein is gluten, the specific name for the protein from wheat, and it is the second and very strong contestant in this group of isolates from agricultural crops.

Processes have been worked out to separate the protein from the starch and then dry it under very special conditions to retain its vitality. It is this unique viscoelastic property, which confers on this material very special performance characteristics not matched in its entirety by any other functional protein, which is so valuable. Although on its own gluten has not a high biological value (it is low in lysine, an essential amino acid), fortification with lysine, now an easily obtainable and cheap amino acid, brings it to the same high standards as meat or casein. Its good taste, its well-proven nutritional qualities and its freedom from metabolic side effects (except in the one case of sufferers from coeliac disease) will make it a valuable companion in protein fortification.

ISOLATES FROM LEGUME AND OILSEED SPECIES

Finally, we have the isolates from the legume and oilseed species, which judging from the state of the art reached at the moment will play the most prominent part in the first generation of novel proteins, with single cell proteins, of which I am going to give you a short account, competing vigorously by the middle of this decade.

It is the soya bean, however, that leads the field at the moment. Of 115 million metric tons of oilseed produced in the world, the USA dominates with 67% and China follows with 28%. It is, therefore, not surprising that many tens of millions of dollars have gone into the research and development of the isolate from this important cash crop.

In our own laboratories, we mounted a considerable research programme into the isolation of a functional protein from the home-grown field or tic bean (*Vicia faba* L.), a legume containing about 24–28% protein, very little fat and the remainder a very useful carbohydrate fraction.

It is these two isolates, from the soya bean or from the British field bean, that are going to play an important part in the manufacture of novel foods. In small percentages, because of their ability to hold meat juices and fat, they are already used in existing food products, such as meat patties, sausages, chilies and a variety of other items, but the isoelectric product (the non-water dispersable one) is destined to be spun into an edible fibre from which meat analogues can be produced. These analogues, poised to enter the market in the near future, are attractive in texture and flavour, having been the subject of many years of research and development studies. In contrast to many medium quality meats, they are tender in bite, very low in fat content and many contain natural meat extracts as flavour.

Another process for forming simulated meats is by thermoplastic die extrusion. A semi-moist plastic proteinaceous mixture is drawn under conditions of high pressure and temperature through an orifice into conditions of lower temperature and pressure. The effect of flash-lowering these conditions results in rapid expansion of the material, yielding a fibrous product. In this process, which is considerably less expensive, there are only three main steps:

1. the preparation of the protein material;
2. the extrusion;
3. the final processing.

The final processing means cutting the emerging ribbon into chunks of various sizes and shapes to simulate meat textures or thin strands, and these chunks and strands can be stored moist under refrigerated conditions or dried and packaged like cereal products.

Rehydration, as with spun analogues, is by immersion in warm water.

The flavour of this type of product is in some cases not quite comparable to that of the spun product but continuous improvements in quality are taking place. Minced meat-type products from this process appear to be particularly acceptable in flavour and texture and are sold in countries like Japan and America and are beginning to be sold here and on the Continent on quite a scale. There is no doubt that the application of a high degree of skill and expertise can give acceptable foods and their quality will steadily improve as the competence of the manufacturers, aided by a considerable research and development effort, increases.

And now, let me quickly cover the area of so-called 'biosynthesised proteins', lumped together now under the generic name of 'single cell protein'—SCP, although many are not true single cell organisms but are multicellular. The organisms involved here are bacteria, yeast, microfungi and algae, grown in most cases on widely different substrates.

ICI grow bacteria (gram-negative (*Pseudomodas*) on methanol, BP grow yeasts on pure or unrefined hydrocarbons and we grow microfungi on carbohydrate substrates. There are pros and cons for each project. In bacteria you have the very tough, thick cell wall, lots of chitinous material,

TABLE 2

ESSENTIAL AMINO ACIDS IN SOME 'SINGLE CELL PROTEINS' COMPARED WITH THE 1957 FAO PROVISIONAL PATTERN

Amino acid	Essential (FAO)	RHM fungal protein	Candida utilis (yeast)	BP protein (yeast)	Esso–Nestle protein (bacteria)	Chlorella (alga)	Spirulina maxima (alga)
Leucine	4·8	7·9	9·1	8·0	5·6	6·8	8·0
Isoleucine	4·2	4·0	6·0	5·2	3·6	3·1	6·0
Valine	4·2	4·3	7·3	5·5	4·5	4·8	6·5
Lysine	4·2	6·0	7·1	7·4	6·5	4·9	4·6
Methionine	2·2 ⎱	2·1	1·6 ⎱	1·7 ⎱	2·0 ⎱	1·4 ⎱	1·4 ⎱
Cystine	2·0 ⎰ 4·2	1·5	0·4 ⎰ 2·0	0·8 ⎰ 2·5	0·6 ⎰ 2·6	0·8 ⎰ 2·2	0·4 ⎰ 1·8
Phenylalanine	2·8	4·0	5·3	5·0	2·9	3·5	5·0
Threonine	2·8	5·1	6·1	5·4	4·0	3·9	4·6
Tyrosine	2·8	3·3	4·3	Not reported	Not reported	2·6	4·0
Tryptophan	1·4	2·2	1·5	1·2	0·9	1·8	1·4
Σ essential	31·4	40·4	47·7	39·2 (+4·0) (43·2)	30·6 (+4·0) (34·6)	32·6	41·9

reduced digestibility, but high nitrogen content. However, this high nitrogen must not be confused with high protein since bacteria, due to their fast growth, have a very high nucleic acid content (20–25 %) which makes them, therefore, unsuitable for human consumption. Yeasts grow more slowly, have a lower nucleic acid content, but have so far persistently produced an allergic factor when tested on humans, resulting in vomiting, diarrhoea or other indications of malabsorption, making this type of product, at this moment, suitable only as animal feed.

In contrast to these organisms, microfungi, which we have screened and after a long screening programme have selected, appear to show none of these disadvantages. A thin cell wall ensures high digestibility; regulated slower growth ensures lower RNA and genetic manipulations have enabled us to produce for the first time a vegetable cell with the amino acid profile of an animal protein. We grow this organism in continuous culture to ensure optimum environmental conditions, maximum controllability (pH, oxygen tension, heat transfer, etc.) and harvest continuously to obtain a biomass of strictly regular composition in quality and quantity, an absolute prerequisite for a material destined for human consumption.

The growth rates of SCP as compared with traditional animal protein are phenomenal. Though nutritional qualities of a product are of vital importance, the first requirement for a food for man is its acceptable texture and flavour. We eat food first and foremost because we enjoy eating it and it is quite useless to have a perfect diet in a form which men will not eat. Incaparina is such an example, fortified rice another. We believe that we have, as food manufacturers, the knowledge and resources to create acceptable foods from this filamentous biomass.

Table 2 shows the essential amino acid composition of some SCPs compared with the 1957 FAO provisional pattern.

We see, in the many products I have described, a distinct and expanding field. Where meat is available at a price people can afford, these new products will not supplant the existing food items but form an alternative in the increasing protein food market, due also to the need to reduce carbohydrate intake to avoid the most obvious form of malnutrition in western society, namely obesity.

BIBLIOGRAPHY

Gray, W. D. (1970). *Crit. Rev. Fd. Technol.*, **1**, No. 2, 225.
Solomons, G. L. and Scammell, G. (1970). British Patent Pending.
Spicer, A. (1971). In *Third International Congress of Food Science and Technology, SOS/70 Proceedings,* p. 296, Institute of Food Technologists, Washington.
Spicer, A. and Solomons, G. L. (1970), British Patent 1210356.

CHAPTER 17

Possible changes in fat consumption in the future

A. T. JAMES

Colworth Welwyn Laboratory, Unilever Limited, Sharnbrook

Whilst there has been much progress in our understanding of fat meta-bolism and clarification of the hyperlipoproteinaemias, the major interest in fats and human nutrition during the last ten years has been attempts at the determination of the connection between the level and nature of dietary fats and the incidence of coronary heart disease. Apart from purely epi-demiological investigations a number of prospective and retrospective studies of humans have been reported together with much work with experimental animals.

In some countries, official and semi-official committees were set up to report on the subject and have either published new reports or updated old ones, the result of which has been a stiffening of views on the subject. Over the next ten years, this will change the pattern of fat intake in the 'advanced' countries.

This paper summarises their conclusions by quoting from their reports.

THE UNITED STATES

The American Heart Association
This organisation, the largest and most influential body in this area in the United States, issued statements on 'diet and heart disease' in 1961 and 1965. In 1967 sufficient additional data had appeared for the Chairman of the AHA Committee on Nutrition to appoint a sub-committee to review the recent literature. This sub-committee reported in the spring of 1968. The full Nutrition Committee then held many sessions revising the initial report; the result was submitted to the Central Committee who after further revision issued in 1968 a new statement which contained the following:

> 'Coronary heart disease is the result of many factors. Diets rich in saturated fat and cholesterol represent one important risk factor which can be safely modified'.

The statement goes on to make the following dietary recommendation for 'healthy' individuals; such recommendations are stated to be particularly applicable to individuals with increased risk as determined by blood lipid levels:

'(a) A calorie intake adjusted to achieve and maintain proper weight. Correction of obesity may reduce elevated serum lipid concentration.

(b) A decrease in the intake of saturated fats, and an increase in the intake of polyunsaturated fats. An intake of less than 40% of calories from fat is considered desirable. Of this total, polyunsaturated fats should probably comprise twice the quantity of saturated fats.

(c) A substantial reduction in cholesterol in the diet. The average daily diet in the United States contains approximately 600 mg cholesterol. Sharp reduction in dietary intake of cholesterol will reduce the concentration of serum cholesterol in most people. In hypercholesterolemic individuals, reduction of dietary cholesterol to less than 300 mg daily is recommended.

In addition, the use of vegetables, cereals, and fruits is suggested to supply most of the dietary carbohydrates and is considered preferable to excessive use of sugar, including candy, soft drinks, and other sweets.'

The United States Inter-Society Commission on Heart Disease Resources
This commission was created through a contract with Regional Medical Programs Service to help fulfil the requirements of Section 907 of Public Law 89–239 which established the Regional Medical Programs in 1965. The commission used two study groups, the Atherosclerosis Study Group and the Epidemiology Study Group. The commission reported in December 1970 ('The Primary Prevention of the Atherosclerotic Diseases') and those parts relevant to this enquiry are quoted below.

'Summary of the possibility of primary prevention
Converging lines of epidemiological, clinical and experimental evidence, both animal and human, support the judgement that the relationship between the risk factors, particularly the major risk factors—*i.e. hypercholesterolemia*, cigarette smoking, hypertension— and the development of coronary heart disease is probably causal.'

'Diet and food modifications
The Commission recommends the following modification of diet for the general public and particularly for individuals with marked increased risk of premature atherosclerosis:

1. calorie intake be adjusted to achieve and maintain optimal weight;
2. reduction of dietary cholesterol to less than 300 mg/day;
3. substantial reduction of dietary saturated fats.

The Commission therefore recommends that the food industry be encouraged by the medical profession and the government and supported by the general public to make available leaner meats and processed meats, dairy products, frozen desserts and baked goods reduced in saturated fats, cholesterol and calories, and visible fats and oils (margarine, shortenings, mayonnaises, salad dressings, oils) of low saturated fat and cholesterol content.'

Under the heading of Fats and Oils the Commission says (our italics):

'Promotion of fats and oils low in saturated fats and cholesterol for table spreads, shortenings, cooking and salad dressings, etc. In some areas of the the country, state and/or local laws prohibit the use of butter substitutes in restaurants and institutions. These laws should be repealed.'

Under the section entitled 'Public and Professional Education', after dealing with the importance of education in nutrition, they say:

'Food manufacturers have an excellent opportunity to provide public education through advertising. They should be encouraged to call attention in their advertising to the type and amount of fat and the cholesterol content of their products.'

Results in the US
1. Such evidence from these powerful medical bodies has resulted in the US Food and Drug Administration relaxing the 12-year-old prohibition of any labelling of the fat content and fat composition of food. They originally suggested mandatory measures but it is now likely that labelling will be voluntary.
2. The US National Academy of Sciences—National Research Council's Food and Nutrition Board has publicly recommended that the Food Industry develop products that will enable consumers to lower their intake of saturated fat and cholesterol relatively easily.

NORWAY, SWEDEN AND FINLAND

Combined medical boards
The Medical Boards of the Scandinavian countries have official responsibilities in their countries somewhat analogous to those of the Surgeon

General of the US Public Health Service in the United States but with authority also in physician licensure and the national hospital systems, as well as the aspects of public health, medical care, and research that come under the jurisdiction of USPHS in the United States. The Boards are non-political and as befits their high responsibility, they act with deliberation after critically reviewing the advice of leading authorities in the matters under consideration. When they act collectively, as in this matter of the diet, the result is particularly authoritative.

On 3 May, 1968 an official collective recommendation on diet in the Scandinavian countries was released at simultaneous press conferences in Oslo, Stockholm, and Helsinki by the Medical Boards of Norway, Sweden and Finland. The report states the following:

> 'In Scandinavia, as in many other countries which are highly developed, eating habits have changed considerably during the twentieth century. The most notable change is a decrease in the total consumption of cereal products and an increase in the total consumption of fats. The consumption of sugar has also risen a great deal since the turn of the century. In the Scandinavian countries, approximately half (45–60 %) of the total calorie requirement is met by fats and sugar. At the beginning of the twentieth century, these two nutritive substances supplied only a third, or less, of the calories.'

Under the section entitled 'Consequences of faulty diets' the statement says:

> 'The importance of diet in causing atherosclerosis has been increasingly seriously considered in recent years. There is a close connection between the development of atherosclerotic cardiovascular diseases and the serum cholesterol level. Middle-aged men with a high serum cholesterol level get atherosclerotic heart disease more often than those who have a low serum cholesterol value. People with an hereditary tendency towards an increase in the serum cholesterol not infrequently develop severe atherosclerosis as early as 30–40 years of age. In population groups with an average low serum cholesterol level, atherosclerotic cardiovascular diseases are less common than in groups with high serum cholesterol levels.
>
> A diet rich in saturated fatty acids has an increasing effect on the serum cholesterol. The consumption of polyunsaturated fatty acids brings about a change in the opposite direction. It has also been discovered that the serum cholesterol rises if one often eats foodstuffs rich in cholesterol. A typical feature of diet in countries with a high prevalence of atherosclerotic diseases is usually that the diet is rich in fat and contains a high proportion of saturated fatty acids and a comparatively small quantity of polyunsaturated fatty acids.'

Under the section entitled 'Desirable changes of diet' they say among other things the following:

'The use of saturated fat should be reduced and the consumption of polyunsaturated fats be increased simultaneously.'

In a final section entitled 'Information on better diets' they make the following statement:

'To carry out the above program, we require the cooperation not only of doctors but of all those who give instruction on questions of nutrition or who are responsible for catering on a large scale, particularly in schools, the military forces, hospitals and similar institutions and other eating places.

It is of pressing importance that the food industry pay attention to the recommendations made here in their choice of raw products and in the manufacture of cooked meats and provisions, other semi-prepared foods and ready-cooked food. The industry ought to specify the contents used in their products in a better way than before.'

Again their conclusions match all those quoted so far.

NEW ZEALAND

In 1969 the Minister of Science in the New Zealand Government asked the Royal Society of New Zealand to set up a committee:

'To make a critical examination of the available information on factors involved in the causation of coronary artery disease, where relevant to consider other detrimental and beneficial effects on human health of substances reported to influence coronary artery disease, and to report on their findings.'

This Committee reported to the Minister on 23 May, 1971, and the full document has only recently been available here. On page 82 the following conclusion is drawn:

'13. With regard to dietary recommendations the Committee concludes that:

(a) So far as the general population is concerned the present stage of knowledge does not justify advising any major changes in dietary habits aimed specifically at reducing the incidence of coronary heart disease. It is considered that this objective can best be achieved by adherence to the type of well-balanced diet which would be advised on general medical grounds for maintenance of good health (*See* also supplementary note).

(b) In particular, aggressive efforts to encourage the New Zealand population to increase the consumption of polyunsaturated fats at the expense of the present normal dietary fats are not justified. Nevertheless the Committee considers that there is a place for making available limited supplies of butter fortified with vegetable oil rich in linoleic acid for medical use in cases of those high coronary risk patients in whom clinical evidence suggests could respond to an increased intake of linoleic acid. This course would appear preferable to the use of linoleic acid-rich cooking oils.

(c) At the same time efforts should be made to minimise cholesterol intake by reducing consumption of cholesterol-risk foods such as eggs and brains. In particular, eggs should be restricted. In making this recommendation it is noted that one egg per day approximately doubles normal cholesterol intake and that two eggs per day cancel the cholesterol-lowering effect of diets designed for this purpose.'

This statement is much less decisive than those quoted previously, but on the following page the document ends with a most interesting 'Supplementary note'. This reads as follows (our italics):

'*Most*, but not all, the members of the Committee consider that for those individuals whose plasma cholesterol levels are high, the following dietary procedures are available:

(a) limitation of foods rich in cholesterol; (b) avoidance of excessive intake of saturated fats and (c) increasing the level of polyunsaturated fatty acids in the diet. Any of these in isolation could be of little value as the effect of saturated fat limitation could be cancelled by an increased intake of eggs. Similarly if dietary intake of saturated fatty acids such as palmitic acid were increased, double the amount of linoleic acid would be required to prevent elevation of cholesterol levels. In a diet designed to reduce the plasma cholesterol, fatty foods containing cholesterogenic saturated fatty acids should be restricted, but not to a degree that would lead to substitution of carbohydrate for fat to maintain calories. Unless the reduction in saturated fat intake is balanced by the addition of polyunsaturated fat, substitution of carbohydrate would induce hypertriglyceridaemia in some individuals with probable associated risk of CHD. More widespread changes in dietary habits could be recommended if individuals were classified on the basis of their plasma cholesterol, triglyceride and lipoprotein patterns. To complete this task for middle-aged men alone would be formidable.

For the population in general it would be prudent to adjust caloric intake to achieve ideal weight using foods that provide the nutritional requirements in terms of essential amino acids, vitamins and minerals. In New Zealand and in a number of other developed countries, fats provide about 40% of the total calories. This could be reduced with advantage towards 30%.

Some members of the Committee feel that until more satisfactory means of measuring stress are developed no firm conclusions should be drawn concerning this risk factor in CHD. On medical grounds there is also some support for making available table spreads with a high content of polyunsaturated fatty acids.'

This supplementary note (from three or four of the five members of the Committee) is in total agreement with all we have said when it is remembered that a large proportion of the susceptible part of the population in the advanced countries have an elevated serum cholesterol.

AUSTRALIA

National Heart Foundation

This organisation has a Standing Subcommittee appointed to 'maintain a continuing review of research developments in the field of diet as related to heart disease'. Two reports have been issued. The first in 1967 reached the verdict of 'not proven' for a connection between diet and heart disease. In 1971, however, after considering the additional evidence received since 1967, the Committee reversed its previous decision and stated the following (our italics):

'The conclusion of the Committee in 1967 was that the evidence did not permit an unequivocal statement that modification of the dietary fat would prevent coronary heart disease, but there was a strong possibility that it would. In view of the very great toll of coronary heart disease in the community, the Committee was of the opinion that such dietary changes were certainly indicated for individuals at high risk, and particularly for those with hyperlipidaemia.

In the past three years, further evidence has been presented which has strengthened the possibility that such dietary modification is beneficial. In the opinion of the Committee, individuals should be advised to reduce high blood lipid levels. The principles involved are: (1) weight reduction when relevant, by caloric restriction; (2) reduction of the cholesterol content of the diet to less than 300 mg/day; (3) the maintenance of a normal total fat content (usually approximately 40% of the calories), *but the substitution of polyunsaturated for saturated fat to achieve a P:S ratio of 1 or greater* (the simple reduction of total fat intake is not usually recommended, as the substitution of carbohydrate to maintain calories may induce hypertriglyceridaemia). The Committee considered two approaches to a community programme for the prevention of coronary heart disease by reduction of high blood lipid levels:

1. To advise the entire community to effect the necessary dietary changes regardless of each individual's blood level on the grounds that (a) measurement of blood levels of cholesterol and triglycerides introduced technical, logistic and financial complications; (b) even those with relatively low blood lipid levels could derive some benefit by lowering them further.

2. To advise the community that each individual should have a regular health check, in the course of which blood lipid levels—particularly cholesterol and triglycerides—should be measured, on the grounds that: (a) the higher the level, the greater would be the need to reduce it and the greater would be the stimulus to do so; (b) such measurements are a guide to dietary or drug therapy in resistant cases and are important in evaluating progress; (c) this definitive approach would avoid changes in the way of life for those individuals who are not at great risk of developing coronary heart disease; (d) the health check offers an opportunity of identifying and dealing with other risk factors, particularly hypertension.

The Committee considered that the second course was more likely to achieve the desired results, and the Foundation has adopted this course as the basis of its community education programme in the dietary prevention of coronary heart disease.'

Again, essentially the same conclusions as all the other review bodies.

INTERNATIONAL

The World Health Organization

The WHO decided that World Health Day 1972 should be devoted to 'Your heart is your health'. In a general message to the world the Director General, Dr M. G. Candau amongst other things said the following:

'Enormous progress has been made in science and technology and important social and economic achievements have been accomplished. Yet health indicators warn us that all is not well with our civilisation and that its harmonious continuation depends to an extent which might surprise some, on the solution of major health problems such as the cardiovascular diseases. The prevention of those diseases will require some far reaching changes in our way of life and in order to make them possible we must be sure that we call upon all the scientific and technical means at our disposal.

We need better nutrition and healthier living habits. Much more concentrated research is necessary to classify the unknowns of atherosclerosis and ischaemic heart disease. Since some predisposing factors are already present in young people, prevention needs to be concentrated on the young adult, and even on the child and adolescent, by promoting their optimum development.'

The detail behind this message was spelled out in a special issue of 'World Health' by Dr M. G. Karvonen. In this article he listed six rules for reducing the risk of coronary heart disease. These rules are:

'1. Stop cigarette smoking.
2. Stop eating too much.
3. Reduce the amounts of saturated fats in the diet. This is achieved by cutting down fat meats and fat meat products (sausages, salami, etc.), dairy fat, and hardened margarine.
4. Avoid egg yolk.
5. Use grain, fruit, vegetables, fish, salad and cooking oils, and new soft margarine.
6. Have your blood pressure checked at least once every five years; if it is too high, stick to the treatment prescribed.'

Karvonen points out:

'Admittedly much still has to be learned until coronary prevention programmes are ripe for integration in individual and public health programmes. Nevertheless, at each stage of the progress of research, everybody must have the right to receive informed advice, even if further results may modify it. The advice in reducing coronary risk is simple.'

SUMMARY

It can be seen that now a number of national and international review bodies accept the following concepts:

1. That raised serum cholesterol levels in the inhabitants of the advanced countries are indicative of an increased risk of coronary heart disease and that such levels should be decreased as soon as possible.
2. That dietary measures to decrease elevated blood lipid levels should either be freely adopted by the public or made freely available to those many people who wish and need to lower their blood lipid levels. Such dietary measures are based on a reduction of saturated fat intake and a full or partial replacement by polyunsaturated fats.

Such widely published views are bound slowly to affect the general public. It is therefore likely that the food industry may need to make available to the general population a range of products fulfilling such aims and that they should assist the public in education on the principles of correct nutrition.

It is extremely unlikely that any one country can afford the enormous cost of the large scale prospective trial necessary to absolutely establish the dietary fat–heart disease relationship. However, shifts in public consumption towards a higher intake of polyunsaturated fats will occur when alternative foodstuffs are available and are publicised, and this in the long run will provide the data confirming or opposing the relationship.

However, it should be borne in mind that there is a tendency to treat all fats of animal origin as if they were identical. There is no doubt that ruminant fats can be altered in composition only by screening the plant unsaturated fats from the action of the hydrogenating systems of the rumen microorganisms. Non-ruminant fats, *e.g.* pork fat, can however be altered and there is a lack of data on the effects of the possible fats on blood lipid levels.

CHAPTER 18

Carbohydrate foods—today and tomorrow

F. WOOD

Development Director, CPC (United Kingdom) Ltd, Esher

We are fortunate to live in that part of the world where people have seldom had to worry about the quantity of food being available to maintain life and limb as distinct from the developing nations who constantly need food for survival. Rather do we now have to worry about the quality of the food we eat than the quantity. More and more we are being exhorted to cut out carbohydrates, to keep off cream and butter, reduce sucrose intake, eliminate salt—the list of prohibitions or warnings seems inexhaustible, not to mention contradictory. In spite of all this, carbohydrates still contribute about a half of our daily diet, and as such occupy a very important part, but contrary to assumptions made for many years, it is now clear that carbohydrates do not all behave metabolically in the same way.

This symposium is being held to focus attention on the problems of today and tomorrow and to review the factors which alter our eating habits—such matters as economics, convenience, travel, as well as nutritional reasons. Convenience foods are a natural development created by the housewife spending less time in the home kitchen, whether this be by choice of leisure activity or by the economic need of the working housewife. As living standards continue to rise, people travel more frequently and farther from home. Thus, for pleasure and convenience, more people eat out in restaurants, snack bars, canteens, roadside grills, etc. and these facilities are multiplying and thriving—all part of the boom which is the food service industry, which, in turn, demands factory preparation of foods to the catering services as well as the retail outlets.

The demand for such preparation of food has itself created many problems for the research worker. Prepared foods will require longer shelf life, flavour stability, replacement of flavours previously produced by long cooking, reconstitution and packaging solutions. In addition to the techniques of deep freezing, dehydration, aseptic canning and sterilisation which have demanded special properties of ingredients, the dietary factors and the growing demands of consumers also affect the choice of ingredients—none more so than in the carbohydrate field. Carbohydrate food is perhaps a misnomer—since very few foods consist solely of carbohydrates; foods rich in carbohydrate would be a more accurate description.

STARCHES

Cereals and roots rich in natural carbohydrates have been man's staple food through the ages. Whilst we are most familiar with wheat, potatoes and rice, other countries have indigenous materials like manioc root, sago palm, sweet potato or yams and natural gums. Less familiar carbohydrates are the modifications of native starches to provide the necessary characteristics for the demands of today and tomorrow. Native starches normally occur in cereal and roots together with variable amounts of protein, salts and cellulose fibre, and as such are either used directly as, for example, wheat in wholemeal bread, barley in brewing, maize in grain whisky, or are separated by wetmilling to recover the native starch in as pure a condition as possible, for example, maize starch (cornflour) and potato starch.

The native starches of maize, potato and tapioca (manihot) are well known as thickeners for food products or for their gelation properties—blancmange. The individual native starches vary considerably in their intrinsic properties due to the ratio of amylose and amylopectin (Knight, 1969). It was found possible by genetic selection to grow maize with very high amylose content or a very high amylopectin content. Both fractions are polymers of anhydrodextrose, amylose essentially linear and amylopectin a branched structure. The internal configuration of starches is a subject for another occasion, but it is necessary to appreciate this to understand the reasons for modifications of native starches. The gelation, thickening and opacity of maize starch, whilst familiar in the household use for gravy thickeners or blancmanges and custards, are not suitable for many other food applications. The starch is therefore modified by chemical or physical treatments.

One treatment consists of simple degradation of the macromolecule—so-called thin boiling starches—to enable increased solids without high viscosity in the manufacture of, for example, Turkish delight, or oxidation of a few side chains in the molecule to interfere with retrogradation to produce a softer gel, and in more recent times, the formation of ester or ether linkages—the so-called cross bonded starches for special uses in frozen foods, sauces, foodstuffs with low pH, condensed soups, fruit pie fillings, etc. (Barber, 1962). Foods which may undergo alternate freezing and thawing with resultant breakdown of the gel and subsequent separation of the liquid phase are rendered satisfactory by the use of waxy starch or an acetylated distarch phosphate of amylopectin.

GUMS

Another example of the need for modification is the use of pregelatinised starches for instant desserts, either alone or mixed with selected gums.

Many gums have marked synergistic effects on starch systems. Wood (1972) suggests that pectins or carageenan/locust bean combinations have interesting properties. The most widely used to date have been alginates and pectins. By adding up to 10% alginate to selected starches with a small amount of calcium salt and a phosphate chelating agent, gels with superior properties are obtained. When using pectin with starch, low methoxyl pectins require calcium, but high methoxyl pectins require the presence of sugar to produce the desired gel. Starch/pectin blends with milk require heating, whereas starch/alginate blends produce gels in the cold. Starch with carageenan has a quicker setting time than starch alone.

SUGARS

The most important carbohydrates other than starches and gums are the sugars. The principal commercial sugars with annual production over 70 million tons are, of course, sucrose (from cane and subsequently from beet) with natural honey and invert sugar (essentially dextrose and laevulose (fructose)) familiar to all.

The hydrolysis of starches (polymers of anhydrodextrose) was first performed by use of acid, heat and subsequent neutralisation. Decolourisation with carbon, produced crystal clear glucose syrup, principally used for sugar confectionery purposes. In the past 20 years tremendous technological achievements have been, and still are being made, using first acid/enzyme and later enzyme/enzyme systems to control the hydrolysis and produce almost any combination of mono-, di-, tri- and higher saccharides (Maiden, 1970).

The alpha amylase enzyme action on starch is essentially one of liquefaction and if followed by beta amylase according to the time and temperature of conversion, the resulting syrup can have a high proportion of maltose. By use of amyloglucosidase (glucamylase), the starch may be converted to essentially dextrose, and with subsequent purification and crystallisation will yield dextrose according to imposed conditions.

The degree of hydrolysis is expressed as the Dextrose Equivalent (DE) and by definition of the Codex recommendation to governments, glucose syrup is an aqueous solution of nutritive saccharide obtained from starch and with a minimum DE of 20 (FAO/WHO, 1969).

Any hydrolysis product below 20 DE is a maltodextrin, whilst pure dextrose is, of course, 99·5 DE minimum.

More recently, due to continued discovery and application of new enzymes, more and more sugars are becoming available.

The most recent development is enzymic production of fructose (laevulose) syrups and crystalline fructose as distinct from traditional invert sugar. Whilst fructose has been naturally available in honey and certain fruits, the development of the enzyme laevulase has allowed the economic production from starch of glucose syrups containing amounts of laevulose valuable as a sweeter syrup (Kooi and Smith, 1972). Fructose is also now being recovered by passing invert syrup through columns of divinylbenzene resin, cross bonded with polystyrene in the presence of calcium ions and separating the dextrose and fructose (Boehringer, 1969).

An alternative technique is to oxidise the dextrose to gluconic acid and separate from fructose as calcium salt. The single or multiple addition of enzymes of order of 0·05 to 0·1% on weight of carbohydrate is being superseded by the use of immobilised enzymes so that one passes the carbohydrate solution through a fixed membrane of enzyme to effect the desired changes and the enzyme can thus be used continuously and without destruction.

The economic production of dextrose, fructose, maltose, xylose, either collectively in syrups, or as individual sugars, allows further developments by hydrogenation.

Dextrose, of course, on hydrogenation yields sorbitol and the hydrogenation of glucose syrups in Sweden received a lot of publicity for anti-cariogenic sweets. Maltose yields maltitol, xylose–xylitol, lactose–lactitol and fructose–mannitol, etc. These, of course, are no longer carbohydrates, but are being actively investigated for diabetic foods, low calorie foods and other specialised applications in place of carbohydrates.

FOODS

Having identified many of the carbohydrates now available as ingredients for foods, let me turn to their uses or projected uses.

The reasons for growth in usage of modern glucose syrups is that they have many important properties apart from sweetness. They are not, therefore, used as an alternative to sucrose or simply to inhibit sucrose crystallisation.

Depending on their composition, a low DE glucose syrup confers humectant control on sugar confectionery by lowering the equilibrium moisture content. By contrast, high DE syrups used in gum and jelly confections retain moisture, increasing the shelf life and improving texture.

Ice cream manufacturers use glucose syrups for their ability to prevent large ice crystals forming and increasing the solids content without excessive sweetness.

Glucose syrups have become standard ingredients in jam and marmalade manufacture by reducing sweetness level whilst maintaining the high solids level to prevent mould growth, and at the same time allowing the fruit flavour to predominate over sweetness.

Reducing sugars have valuable properties including Maillard reactions with proteins, allowing development of caramel colour in baking products. Caramel is manufactured by Maillard reactions and is extensively used in Cola drinks, vinegars, spirits, etc.

In canning of fruit, the use of glucose syrup together with sucrose has proved extremely valuable in providing the requisite body and mouth feel of the cut out syrup without excessive sweetness. In the canning of grapefruit in California the two sugars are varied to counteract the degree of sweetness during extended harvesting. The soft drink industry also makes use of glucose syrups.

The brewing industry requires readily fermentable as well as slowly fermentable sugars, and syrups are now manufactured to the same profile as natural wort syrups.

With the proliferation of new enzyme systems previously referred to, it is not difficult to see how it is now possible to extend the use of glucose syrups by controlling the profile of sugars present. It is now possible to produce boiled sweets, for example, solely from glucose syrup and to eliminate sucrose entirely, if this was found to be desirable.

Fructose and fructose syrups are relatively new and readily available, but still expensive in relation to other sugars. Recent claims that fructose is insulin independent and therefore of value to diabetics are by no means proved to medical experts. A recent symposium held in Helsinki (January, 1972) has published a comprehensive survey of current research in the metabolism of fructose (Nikkilä and Huttunen, 1972).

Maltose rich syrups allow considerable reduction in sucrose content of boiled sweets and have been the subject of comparative research in reducing dental caries.

The term maltodextrins is not new—simple acid conversions to 15–20 DE have been utilised in certain dry baby foods for generations, but today a whole range of selected maltodextrins from 3 DE to 19 DE are available as powders. They form the basis of products like coffee whiteners and are used as flavour encapsulators. Their main advantages are water solubility and almost complete lack of sweetness. Liquids which, on spray drying, normally produce an hygroscopic powder, when spray dried with maltodextrins produce free flowing powders.

Two other factors which influence the demand for newly available carbohydrates are those of legislation and medical research. The harmonisation of the world food laws in the past decade by FAO/WHO—the Codex Alimentarius—and the need for harmonisation of food laws within the EEC are creating approval for the use of certain modified starches and sugars. Many countries' laws had become antiquated and restricted sugar to sucrose only, because, when they were approved originally, sucrose was the commonly available carbohydrate. Approval in the case of Codex and EEC both demand extensive and satisfactory toxicological testing.

Medical research and literature obviously influence the ultimate choice of carbohydrate—perhaps the best known examples being the present controversy on the effects of excess sucrose consumption and the revived subject of fibre (another carbohydrate) and diverticular disease (Burkitt, 1972).

The comparative cariogenicity of carbohydrates is also fascinating and whilst it may well be much too late for many of the present generation, hopefully the work with the 'artificial mouth' (Wilson, 1970) will point the way to allow the future generations at least to dig their graves with their *own* teeth.

REFERENCES

Barber, G. A. (1962). *Modification on Starch for Industrial Use*, SCI Monograph 16.

Boehringer, C. F. (1969). US Patent 3483031.

Burkitt, D. P. (1972). *Br. Nutr. Fdn. Bull.*, No. 7, 29.

FAO/WHO (1969). Codex Standards CAC/RS.9.

Knight, J. W. (1969). *The Starch Industry*, Pergamon Press, Oxford.

Kooi, E. R. and Smith, R. S. (1972). *Food Tech.*, **26**, No. 9, 51.

Maiden, A. M. (1970). In *Glucose Syrups and Related Carbohydrates*, edited by G. G. Birch, L. F. Green and C. B. Coulson, p. 3, Applied Science, London.

Nikkilä, E. A. and Huttunen, J. K. (1972). Clinical and metabolic aspects of fructose, *Acta med. scand.*, Supp. 542.

Wilson, R. F. (1970). *J. dent Res.*, **49**, 180.

Wood, F. (1972). *Gelation Properties of Starch Systems*, BFMIRA Symposium 13.

CHAPTER 19

Non-assimilable components of food

D. A. T. SOUTHGATE

Dunn Nutritional Laboratory, Cambridge

Non-assimilable components are by definition not absorbed into the body and therefore appear in the faeces either unchanged or in a modified form. Under certain conditions, however, most dietary constituents can be found in the faeces, and it is useful to consider briefly the processes involved in digestion and absorption in order to identify the various conditions under which a dietary constituent may not be assimilated.

The various stages in digestion and absorption are presented schematically in Fig. 1. The terms intake, digestion, secretion, absorption and flow may be considered to have the dimension of mass per unit time; these

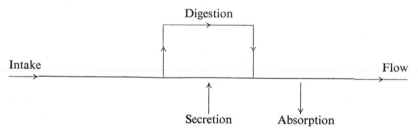

Fig. 1. *Schematic representation of the processes involved in assimilation.*

terms are therefore rates. It is possible to distinguish the various conditions leading to the appearance of a dietary component in the faeces. This will occur when the rate of absorption is lower than the rates of intake, digestion or flow through the absorptive regions of the tract. In addition, where a component must be digested before absorption can occur it will also appear in the faeces when the rate of digestion is less that the rate of intake.

The situations where dietary constituents are not assimilated can be classified, albeit arbitrarily, according to their primary cause (Table 1).

The first two can be considered as being pathological in origin, arising first when flow through the tract exceeds the absorptive capacity as a result of infection or irritation of the tract, leading to the appearance in the faeces of dietary constituents which are usually well absorbed or products

derived from them. The second occurs when the rate of digestion or
absorption is reduced because a digestive or absorptive enzyme or other
secretion is deficient. This is the case in the various carbohydrate intoler-
ances and steatorrhoea.

Under the heading 'physiological' I have considered the situation where
intake exceeds either the digestive or absorptive capacity of the tract for
purely quantitative reasons. For most dietary constituents which are well
absorbed effects of this nature are rarely observed. Wollaeger *et al.* (1947),
for example, found that in adults the intake of fat had to be increased to

TABLE 1

CLASSIFICATION OF THE TYPES OF NON-ASSIMILATION

Primary cause	*Classification*
Gastrointestinal infection	
Lack of specific enzymes or other secretions due to congenital or other causes	Pathological
Overloading of absorptive or digestive capacity	Physiological
Interaction between dietary components	Dietary
Ingestion of dietary components in an insoluble or indigestible form	Dietary/physiological

150–200 g/day before there was any marked increase in the faecal excretion
of fat. Masterton *et al.* (1957) similarly found little evidence for increased
faecal excretion of fat on high fat intakes and various overfeeding studies
such as those of Miller and Mumford (1967) have usually failed to demonstrate any impairment in assimilation on greatly increased intakes.

In young infants there is some evidence for an effect of this sort
(Southgate *et al.*, 1969); for the faecal excretion of fat increases in an
exponential fashion as fat intake rises, suggesting that the limiting rate of
absorption is being approached.

There are two cases where the cause is primarily of dietary origin; the
first occurs when constituents in the diet interact to form substances which
cannot be absorbed. This is most frequently observed for inorganic
constituents such as calcium or iron which react with various anions such
as phosphate, oxalate or phytate to form insoluble compounds which are
poorly absorbed. A second type, primarily dietary in origin, depends on
the form in which the constituents are ingested. In a sense it is also
physiological because the endogenous secretions do not contain the
appropriate enzymes for the digestion and absorption of these substances.
These are truly non-assimilable components of the diet.

While faeces contain nitrogenous materials there is no convincing
evidence that there are specific proteins which are non-assimilable by the

normal subject; pieces of cartilage can be recovered from faeces on occasion but these are usually exceptional. The same can be said for lipids although there is some evidence that long-chain saturated fatty acids are less well assimilated than either unsaturated acids or those of shorter chain length.

One must, however, be cautious when interpreting the results of faecal analysis and relating the results obtained to dietary intake. This caution is necessary because of the high concentrations of microorganisms in the large intestine and rectum. These organisms use as their growth medium the mixture leaving the small intestine and this growth is accompanied by a great variety of changes during the passage from the small intestine to the colon in the components which have not been absorbed. Aylward and Woods (1962) showed that the faecal lipids were considerably more saturated than the dietary lipid; which could be interpreted as showing that the saturated fatty acids were less well absorbed. However, it is also consistent with the known properties of the intestinal flora and its environment which would favour hydrogenation of the unsaturated fatty acids.

The non-assimilable components of the diet are listed in Table 2. This

TABLE 2

NON-ASSIMILABLE DIETARY COMPONENTS

Inorganic	Components ingested in an insoluble or potentially insoluble form
Organic	Mineral oils (usually contaminants)
	Waxes
	Gums
	Structural carbohydrates of the plant cell wall
	Lignin
	Modified carbohydrates
	Algal polysaccharides
	Some food additives, dyes, etc.

list is by no means complete but shows the great range of types of substance involved. Many of these are eaten in very small amounts and are concentrated in the faeces. Faecal material is a complex mixture of living and dead bacteria and their metabolites, the structural materials of the plant cell wall, proteins and lipids from the diet or endogenous secretions together with a range of pigments, plant waxes, many food additives, insoluble salts and traces of mineral oil.

The measurement of the remnants of the endogenous secretions is extremely difficult, as is the fractionation of faecal material into substances of dietary or bacterial origin (Trémolières et al., 1960).

DIETARY FIBRE

Quantitatively the most important group of non-assimilable components in the diet are the substances found in the plant cell wall. This is composed of a number of types of compounds mainly of a polysaccharide nature. The actual composition of the wall varies during the course of its development, the primary wall being made up of cellulose fibrils laid down as a network on a middle lamella rich in pectic substances (Wardrop, 1962).

As the cell matures, increasing amounts of cellulose are formed on this primary wall; the fibrils are, however, laid down in a regular fashion and deposited in a matrix of so-called hemicellulose (Muhlethaler, 1961). Hemicellulose itself is a complex mixture of a number of different types of polysaccharide including arabino-xylans, galactans and polyuronans. As the wall matures the non-carbohydrate lignin is deposited within the matrix. Lignin is a complex substance formed by the condensation of coniferyl and other plant alcohols and forms a two-dimensional net or three-dimensional matrix within the wall starting at the exterior of the wall. By the time the wall is completely lignified the cell itself is dead.

These substances collectively make up the fraction 'dietary fibre' which can be defined as the polysaccharides which are not hydrolysed by endogenous secretions of the digestive tract, or alternatively, the unavailable carbohydrates, and lignin. The distinction between dietary fibre and the empirically measured crude fibre is illustrated in Fig. 2.

Total carbohydrate 'by difference'
- Sugars ⎫
- Dextrins ⎬ Available carbohydrate
- Starches ⎭
- ·Pectins ⎫
- Crude fibre[a] { Hemicelluloses / Celluloses / Lignin } ⎬ Unavailable carbohydrate[b] ≡ Dietary fibre

[a] This fraction may include small amounts of hemicellulose.

[b] As originally defined this included the non-carbohydrate lignin.

Fig. 2. Distinction between crude fibre and dietary fibre.

In most western communities highly lignified plant tissues are rarely eaten in large amounts and are usually discarded during the preparation of the food. The crude fibre content of the diet and its dietary fibre content is usually therefore low compared with that of the diet eaten in other parts of the world. Crude fibre alone is often not a good measure of the total amount of non-assimilable carbohydrates in the diet. For example, where the plantain banana is the staple food the intake of dietary fibre would be quite high whereas that of crude fibre would be low.

The effects of increasing the intake of 'dietary fibre' on faecal excretion are quite striking. There is an increase in the weight of faeces passed and the stools contain more water probably due to the water-binding properties of the hemicelluloses. The unavailable carbohydrates also provide a substrate which promotes the growth of microorganisms in the large intestine. Williams and Olmsted (1936) showed that the hemicellulose fraction was responsible for the major part of this increase in stool weight principally due to its use as a substrate by the intestinal microflora.

The combined effects result in a bulky, moister mass in the large intestine which appears to stimulate peristalsis and usually leads to a reduced transit time through the gastrointestinal tract.

In the last two years considerable evidence has been produced which indicates that dietary fibre forms an essential part of the human diet and that its deficiency is one of the causes of many diseases in western communities especially those concerning the large intestine (Painter and Burkitt, 1971). Low intakes of dietary fibre have also been implicated in coronary heart disease and diabetes (Trowell, 1972).

This leads to the question posed in the title of this session, how much dietary fibre should one consume?

In the 1930s there was a considerable interest in the laxative effects of wheat bran and the unavailable carbohydrates from a variety of vegetable sources. Cowgill and Anderson (1932) on the basis of studies with wheat bran eaten by a group of young men, came to the conclusion that a minimum intake of 90–100 mg of crude fibre/kg bodyweight/day was required to achieve normal laxation rates.

Robertson (1972) has estimated the crude fibre intakes in the United Kingdom using total food supply data, and her calculations suggest that the average intakes were around 4 to 5 g/head/day which is equivalent to some 10 to 15 g/head/day of dietary fibre.

Analyses of a composite of the average diet eaten in the USA gave a value of 6 g/head/day of crude fibre and 19 g/head/day of unavailable carbohydrate and lignin.

Using Cowgill and Anderson's minimum requirements and an average bodyweight of 65 kg it would appear that the average diet eaten in both the United Kingdom and the USA provides only the minimum amount required for normal functioning of the large intestine, and the average consumption data conceal the range of individual variations of intake which occur in the population.

The bases for these deductions, however, are not as firm as one would wish, being based on a very limited amount of experimental data. Much more information of both a qualitative and quantitative nature is required concerning the nature of dietary fibre in the human diet coupled with work which will lead to an understanding of the physiological role of these substances in the large intestine and the gastrointestinal tract in general.

REFERENCES

Aylward, F. and Woods, P. D. S. (1962). *Br. J. Nutr.*, **16,** 345.

Cowgill, G. R. and Anderson, W. E. (1932). *J. Am. med. Ass.*, **98,** 1866.

Masterton, J. P., Lewis, H. E. and Widdowson, E. M. (1957). *Br. J. Nutr.*, **11,** 346.

Miller, D. S. and Mumford, P. (1967). *Am. J. clin. Nutr.*, **20,** 1212.

Muhlethaler, K. (1961). In *The Cell*, edited by J. Brachet & A. E. Minsky, Vol. 2, pp. 85–134, Academic Press, New York.

Painter, N. S. and Burkitt, D. P. (1971). *Br. med. J.*, **2,** 450.

Robertson, J. (1972). *Nature, Lond.*, **238,** 290.

Southgate, D. A. T., Widdowson, E. M., Smits, B. J., Cooke, W. T., Walker, C. H. M. and Mathers, N. P. (1969). *Lancet*, **1,** 487.

Trémolières, J., Carre, L., Sautier, C., Faude-May, F., Farquet, J. and Flament, C. (1960). *Annls Nutr. (Paris)*, **14,** 225.

Trowell, H. C. (1972). *Am. J. clin. Nutr.*, **25,** 926.

Wardrop, A. B. (1962). *Botan. Rev.*, **28,** 241.

Williams, R. D. and Olmsted, W. H. (1936). *J. Nutr.*, **11,** 533.

Wollaeger, E. E., Comfort, M. W. and Osterberg, A. E. (1947). *Gastroenterology*, **9,** 272.

CHAPTER 20

Fortification of food with iron—is it necessary or effective?

SHEILA T. CALLENDER

*Nuffield Department of Clinical Medicine,
The Radcliffe Infirmary, Oxford*

Iron deficiency is widespread throughout the world, particularly in those sections of the population whose physiological needs are greatest. In the United Kingdom improvements in nutrition and better access to medical care have reduced the very high incidence found in surveys in the poorer sections of the population during the 1930s, nevertheless various recent studies still show an incidence of overt iron deficiency in 10–20% of adult women and 2–8% of men (Kilpatrick, 1971). The incidence is somewhat higher in both sexes over 75 years of age (McLennan *et al.*, 1973). In Oxford, as part of another study, we examined the blood of 258 healthy adult subjects most of whom were visitors to patients in hospital. Blood relatives of the patients were excluded. Sixteen were found to have a haemoglobin of less than 12 g/100 ml with an iron deficiency type of picture; all were women, giving an incidence of just over 11% in the 142 women in the survey. No attempt was made to determine the frequency of latent iron deficiency but from the studies of McFarlane *et al.* (1967), in a general practice in Glasgow, at least twice as many would be expected to have evidence of latent deficiency with lack of iron stores.

Iron deficiency may fairly readily be defined in laboratory terms, for example by the standards set by the WHO (1968). For the detection of latent iron deficiency it is necessary to measure in addition the plasma iron and the percentage saturation of the iron binding protein or to assess the storage iron by examining the bone marrow for stainable iron. Another and probably the most sensitive test of iron status is the absorption from a standard dose of radioactive iron.

However, having detected iron deficiency in a population, it is quite another matter to determine how important it is in relation to morbidity. A number of workers have shown that haemoglobin levels down to about 8 g/100 ml may give rise to little apparent disability, and although an increase in haemoglobin may be obtained in response to iron therapy, most observers have failed to show any significant accompanying improvement in symptoms when compared with the results of placebo treatment (Elwood and Wood, 1966; Morrow *et al.*, 1968).

This does not necessarily mean that moderate anaemia results in no physical disability. In relation to this it is perhaps interesting to note that in Oxford of 5597 new female blood donors recruited in one year only 85 were rejected at their first visit on the grounds of anaemia (Grant, personal communication), that is about one tenth of the number expected from our study of randomly selected women from the same area. There are obviously a number of reasons why women may volunteer to be blood donors but one of them is at least likely to be physical wellbeing.

A more definite relationship between minor degrees of anaemia and physical fitness has been shown in a group of agricultural workers in Guatemala where a highly significant correlation was found between haematocrit value and physical fitness as measured by a step test in subjects with haematocrits of 35% and over (Viteri and Cifuentes, 1973). This suggests that minor degrees of iron deficiency are an indication of suboptimal health, as does the fact that about one third of women with latent iron deficiency who are followed up for over two years will develop overt deficiency (McFarlane *et al.*, 1967).

If it is accepted that the presence of iron deficiency is not ideal how far can it be attributed to nutritional deficiency?

In infancy the development of iron deficiency is almost inevitable if feeding exclusively with breast milk or cows' milk is unduly prolonged. This is one area in which food iron fortification is manifestly successful. An intake of about 10 mg a day from proprietary milk and infant cereals fortified with iron has been shown convincingly to prevent anaemia in infants (Moe, 1963). Vitamin C is also added to these foods, which is an important factor in promoting efficient absorption.

The case for iron deficiency anaemia in adults being largely attributable to nutritional deficiency and amenable to supplementation is less well founded. Surprisingly, perhaps, studies in which dietary iron intake has been related to the occurrence of iron deficiency anaemia have not shown any clear correlation between low intake and iron deficiency (McLennan *et al.*, 1973).

The present type of Western diet provides about 6 mg iron/1000 kcal (4·2 MJ). Adult men need only to absorb about 1 mg or less of iron per day in order to stay in balance whereas normal women need about twice this amount. From all we know about the physiological requirements of menstruation and pregnancy (Rybo, 1973) it is clear that in women this balance is often precarious; hence prophylactic iron treatment has been widely adopted for pregnant women. In the non-pregnant adult woman, however, it is rare, except perhaps in the case of vegetarians, not to find either an abnormal physiological loss, *i.e.* menorrhagia, or some pathological cause for iron deficiency. It is therefore questionable whether fortification of food with iron could reduce the incidence of iron deficiency.

The problem is certainly complex. The proportion of iron absorbed does not depend on the total iron content of the diet but varies considerably with the composition of the diet especially with regard to the proportion of non-haem and haem iron present. The absorption of the former is influenced by other factors such as phytates, phosphates or the consumption of eggs which inhibit absorption or ascorbic acid which enhances it. Haem iron is independent of such factors and is therefore more efficiently absorbed. The absorption from both haem and non-haem iron is, however, enhanced by the presence of meat protein and therefore meat assumes great importance in the maintenance of positive iron balance, and vegetarians are more prone to iron deficiency (Martinez-Torres and Layrisse, 1973).

If attempts are to be made to increase the average intake of iron, foods chosen for fortification should be cheap and widely used, hence the choice of cereals; but all the studies using biologically labelled foods and foods to which tracer amounts of radioactive iron have been added in the cooking process, have shown poor absorption of iron from cereal products (Elwood *et al.*, 1968; Callender and Warner, 1968; Martinez-Torres and Layrisse, 1973).

In some of our own studies subjects were given a whole, small loaf of either white bread labelled with radioactive iron added to bring the level back to 80% extraction flour or wholemeal bread made with flour labelled biologically. Each subject used the loaf as the sole source of bread until it was completely consumed, and retention of iron from the loaf was measured 10–14 days later (Callender and Warner, 1971). From these studies we made some estimates of the contribution of bread to the daily iron balance in the United Kingdom. This appeared to be no more than 0·1–0·15 mg in normal subjects. Iron deficient subjects might be expected to absorb about twice this amount.

In America for many years iron has been added to bring the content of white bread back to that of wholemeal bread, *i.e.* 3·5 mg/100 g of bread. This has been insufficient to reduce the incidence of iron deficiency and it is now proposed to increase the iron content to 40 mg/pound of flour or 5·5 mg/100 g of bread (Council on Foods and Nutrition, 1972; Finch and Monsen, 1972).

There are considerable technical difficulties in reaching this level of supplementation without deterioration of the flour, the most suitable preparations for the purpose tending to be less soluble and hence less well absorbed.

Cook *et al.* (1973) have studied the availability of radioactive iron from bread rolls with this new level of supplementation. Both iron added as sodium iron pyrophosphate and as ferric orthophosphate was poorly absorbed relative to that added as ferrous sulphate, but 'reduced iron' of particle size 5–10 μ was as well absorbed as ferrous sulphate (8·6% and 9·1% respectively). In the same subjects the mean absorption from a

208 SHEILA T. CALLENDER

reference standard dose of ferrous ascorbate was 34·5 %, *i.e.* the iron in the rolls was about a quarter as well absorbed as the same amount of ferrous iron given alone.

When bread rolls labelled with ^{59}Fe ferrous sulphate were given as a part of a meal together with meat the absorption was again about a quarter of that from the reference standard, but when given without meat it was only about one tenth of that from the iron salt alone.

TABLE 1

ESTIMATED ABSORPTION OF IRON IN UK IF SUPPLEMENTED
TO USA STANDARD

	oz/person/ week	mg Fe/day	mg Fe absorbed with meat	mg Fe absorbed without meat
Bread (all kinds)	34·68	7·7	0·55	0·16
Buns, cakes, biscuits	10·72	2·2	0·16	0·05
Flour	5·39	1·9	0·13	0·04
Total		11·8	0·84	0·25

Data for intake for third quarter 1972 supplied by Ministry of Agriculture, Fisheries and Food.

In the third quarter of 1972, as shown in Table 1, the consumption of bread in this country averaged 34·68 oz/person/week, of flour 5·39 oz/person/week, and of biscuits, cake, etc. 10·72 oz/person/week (Ministry of Agriculture, Fisheries and Food, 1973). This at the American level of supplementation would contribute 11·8 mg of iron/day and from the data of Cook *et al.* (1973) an overall absorption of about 0·84 mg provided meat was taken at each meal. If little or no meat was consumed or eggs were included in the diet the absorption would be far less than this. This estimate, however, does not take into consideration the different consumption by men and women, and women, especially figure conscious young women who are in the vulnerable age group, are likely to consume much less bread and flour products and the men more. A fortification programme, therefore, even at the level suggested in the USA cannot be expected to do more than prevent some women who are marginally deficient from developing overt deficiency.

Further support for the view that fortification of cereals alone is unlikely to be helpful in the prevention of iron deficiency comes from countries where iron deficiency is found notwithstanding a high dietary iron intake. For example a recent study in five villages in southern Iran (Haghshenass *et al.*, 1972) showed that 30 % of children, 24 % of females and 7 % of males over the age of 16 had an anaemia with a haemoglobin less than 12 g/100 ml which responded to iron therapy in spite of the fact that they had a mean daily iron intake of 44·4 mg. This iron was largely derived from the basic food tanok, an unleavened wholemeal wheat bread with a mean iron content of 22 mg/100 g.

Even more striking is the situation in Ethiopia where some of the highest dietary intakes of iron in the world are found. There the staple food is teff and intakes may amount to 500 mg iron/day. About a quarter of the iron is in the grain itself and the rest comes from contamination. Although iron deficiency is infrequent, except in infants, iron overload is also seldom seen in this population and examination of the storage iron in individuals dying from trauma has shown no difference from that found in a comparable Swedish population (Hofvander, 1968).

Apart from the doubt that fortification of cereals with iron could be an effective means of prevention of iron deficiency, considerable anxiety has been expressed about the possible harmful effects of programmes of iron fortification (Crosby, 1970; Conrad, 1972). Iron deficiency is a relatively harmless state compared with iron overload which may lead to widespread damage to the pancreas, liver and heart and is potentially lethal. Furthermore, by the time the iron overload is clinically recognisable much of the damage has already been done.

Deliberate increase in dietary iron by fortification might contribute a hazard in subjects with idiopathic haemochromatosis who lack the normal mechanism for regulating absorption of iron from the gut. Patients with cirrhosis of the liver may also be at risk since some show an inappropriate increase in iron absorption (Callender and Malpas, 1963).

In normal subjects the regulatory mechanism of iron absorption is such that it seems improbable that normal males would suffer any harmful effects from an increase in iron intake. Dietary iron overload certainly can occur in otherwise normal individuals but only in exceptional circumstances, for example in the Bantu where the high dietary intake is derived from the home brewed alcoholic beverages which are prepared in iron pots. The iron is in a soluble form and as much as 2–3 mg/day may be absorbed (Charlton et al., 1973). Iron overload is also prevalent in parts of northern Italy and is associated with the high iron content of the local wine (Perman, 1967).

In conclusion, I do not think the case for further fortification of food with iron in the United Kingdom is very strong. In the prevention of the iron deficiency of infancy it is effective and should be encouraged, but for the reasons I have discussed iron fortification of cereals is unlikely to improve, more than very marginally, the iron balance in adults and it is theoretically possible that it would be hazardous to the small minority of subjects suffering from iron storage diseases such as idiopathic haemochromatosis.

I would prefer to see the problem approached differently. There is a place for food education with emphasis on the importance of meat and citrus fruits in promoting iron absorption. The public should also be made more aware of the hazard of indiscriminate use of analgesics such as aspirin in producing blood loss.

Menorrhagia and gastrointestinal bleeding are by far the most important causes of iron deficiency and the better recognition, for example, of excessive menstrual loss, and its treatment by oral contraceptives or anti-fibrinolytic agents, might well have a far greater effect in reducing the incidence of iron deficiency than any dietary fortification programme.

REFERENCES

Callender, S. T. and Malpas, J. (1963). *Br. med. J.*, **2**, 1516.
Callender, S. T. and Warner, G. T. (1968). *Am. J. clin. Nutr.*, **21**, 1170.
Callender, S. T. and Warner, G. T. (1971). *Haematologica*, **5**, 369.
Charlton, R. W., Bothwell, T. H. and Seftel, H. C. (1973). *Clinics in Haematology*, **2**, 383.
Conrad, M. E. (1972). *J. Am. med. Ass.*, **221**, 408.
Cook, J. D., Minnich, V., Moore, C. V., Rasmussen, A., Bradley, W. B. and Finch, C. A. (1973). In press.
Council on Foods and Nutrition (1972). *J. Am. med. Ass.*, **220**, 855.
Crosby, W. H. (1970). *Archs intern. Med.*, **126**, 911.
Elwood, P. C. and Wood, M. M. (1966). *Br. J. prev. soc. Med.*, **20**, 172.
Elwood, P. C., Newton, D., Eakins, J. D. and Brown, D. A. (1968). *Am. J. clin. Nutr.*, **21**, 1162.
Finch, C. A. and Monsen, E. R. (1972). *J. Am. med. Ass.*, **219**, 1462.
Haghshenass, M., Mahloudji, M., Reinhold, J. G. and Mohammadi, N. (1972). *Am. J. clin. Nutr.*, **25**, 1143.
Hofvander, Y. (1968). *Acta med. scand.*, Suppl. 494.
Kilpatrick, G. S. (1971). In *Iron Deficiency*, edited by L. Hallberg, H.-G. Harworth and A. Vannotti, p. 441, Academic Press, London.
Martinez-Torres, C. and Layrisse, M. (1973). *Clinics in Haematology*, **2**, 339.
McFarlane, D. B., Pinkerton, P. H., Dagg, J. H. and Goldberg, A. (1967). *Br. J. Haemat.*, **13**, 790.
McLennan, W. J., Andrews, G. R., Macleod, C. and Caird, F. I. (1973). *Q. Jl. Med.*, **42**, 1.
Ministry of Agriculture, Fisheries and Food (1973). *Trade and Industry*, 4 January.
Moe, P. J. (1963). *Acta paediat. Stockh*, Suppl. 150.
Morrow, J. J., Dagg, J. H. and Goldberg, A. (1968). *Scott. medical J.*, **13**, 78.
Perman, G. (1967). *Acta med. scand.*, **182**, 281.
Rybo, G. (1973). *Clinics in Haematology*, **2**, 269.
Viteri, F. E. and Cifuentes, E. (1973). In press, quoted by L. Garby (1973). *Clinics in Haematology*, **2**, 245.
WHO (1968). *Tech. Rep. Ser.*, No. 405, 9.

CHAPTER 21

Calcium and vitamin D requirement

B. E. C. NORDIN

Director, Medical Research Council Mineral Metabolism Unit, Leeds

EXPERIMENTAL OBSERVATIONS

Any consideration of the requirement of vitamin D and calcium (or of any other nutrient for that matter) must take into account the clinical effect of a deficiency of these nutrients. Experimental observations in animals going back over many years make it clear that experimental calcium deficiency reduces the amount of bone (particularly trabecular bone) without altering its chemical composition, a condition comparable to clinical osteoporosis in man. Vitamin D deficiency on the other hand produces rickets in the growing animal or osteomalacia in the adult, conditions associated with a reduction in the relative ash content of the bones (Nordin, 1960).

The reason why vitamin D deficiency and calcium deficiency produce these different effects is really outside the scope of the present paper, but can be briefly recapitulated. In essence, it appears that simple calcium deficiency results in an increase in bone resorption, almost certainly mediated through the parathyroid glands (Jowsey and Raisz, 1968), which allows the plasma calcium concentration to be maintained at the expense of the skeleton. Although parathyroid stimulation must occur on a low calcium diet, it does not appear to be of sufficient magnitude to reduce the tubular reabsorption of phosphate or the plasma phosphate concentration. Because the plasma calcium and phosphate concentrations remain essentially unchanged, the mineralisation of new bone is not affected and the ash content of the bones remain normal. (The removal of mineral from the skeleton to maintain the plasma calcium does not affect the ash content of the bones because parathyroid hormone-induced bone resorption always removes matrix and mineral simultaneously.)

Vitamin D deficiency on the other hand lowers the plasma calcium and/or phosphorus levels with the result that the mineralisation of new bone is delayed and the clinical picture of rickets or osteomalacia develops. The most likely explanation for this difference between the effects of calcium and vitamin D deficiency is that the mechanism whereby parathyroid hormone maintains the plasma calcium is itself dependent upon an adequate supply of vitamin D. Parathyroid hormone normally maintains the plasma calcium by its simultaneous actions on calcium absorption in the gastrointestinal tract, on bone resorption and on the tubular reabsorption of calcium in the kidney. Vitamin D is required for the bone resorbing action of parathyroid hormone (Rasmussen and Arnaud, 1967) so that in vitamin D deficiency the plasma calcium falls significantly and the parathryoid glands are stimulated.

This in turn reduces the tubular reabsorption of phosphate and lowers the plasma phosphate concentration. In addition, vitamin D deficiency almost certainly reduces phosphate absorption which contributes further to the hypophosphataemia. Thus in vitamin D deficiency the plasma calcium and/or phosphate levels are reduced in a manner that does not occur in simple calcium deficiency. Vitamin D deficiency therefore gives rise to rickets or osteomalacia whereas simple calcium deficiency only produces osteoporosis.

With these considerations in mind it is possible to discuss the calcium and vitamin D requirement of humans.

CALCIUM REQUIREMENT

Childhood
It is not possible to establish the calcium requirement of children by a simple balance technique because the growing child must be in positive calcium balance and the degree of positive calcium balance which is desirable at different ages is unknown. Nonetheless, various attempts have been made to do so by estimating the effect of calcium intake on calcium retention. The outcome of such studies (reviewed by Sherman, 1952) was that calcium retention in children tended to increase with calcium intake up to an intake of about 1 g/day or even more, and it was on the basis of these observations that the United States National Research Council recommended calcium allowances for children up to 1·4 g/day. The subject was reviewed by Leitch and Aitken (1959) who showed that the calculated addition of calcium to the skeleton during growth rose from about 100 mg daily in early childhood to a peak of about 350 mg daily in early adolescence. In estimating the calcium requirement from these figures they did not, however, allow adequately for the relatively small proportion of dietary calcium that is absorbed and they concluded that existing calcium allowance recommendations were too high. If one assumes that faecal calcium is about 50% of intake and that obligatory calcium loss in the urine is 50 mg (both of these being conservative estimates) one would have to conclude that the calcium requirement during childhood rises from about 250 mg daily at the age of 4 years to about 850 mg daily at the age of 14. These conservative estimates would of course be *mean* estimates of requirement and the allowance should be greater than the

mean requirement to allow for individual variation. Yet the amount recommended by the British panel on dietary allowances is 500 mg daily through early childhood rising to 700 mg around puberty. The latter allowance is probably much less than most adolescent children are actually getting and is presumably meant to imply that the present calcium intake in this country is unnecessarily high.

This is not to suggest that children on inadequate calcium intakes would necessarily develop osteoporosis. It is probable that the intake would have to be very low indeed for this to happen. The most likely effect of sub-optimum intakes of calcium in children is retarded growth. The evidence for this has been reviewed elsewhere (Nordin, 1973) and rests essentially on the following points. First, the increase in height of British school-children during this century has been associated with a proportionately much greater increase in the intake of calcium than of energy or protein. Secondly, milk supplements have been shown to have a very significant effect on growth, such supplements of course providing a much greater addition to dietary calcium intake than to the intake of any other nutrient with the possible exception of riboflavin. Thirdly, 15-year-old Japanese schoolchildren have gained about four inches in the past 15 years during which time dietary calcium intake in Japan has risen from 200 to 600 mg daily and calcium-fortified bread and milk supplements have been issued to the schools. It is of interest that Sherman (1952) showed that restriction of calcium intake in growing rats had a marked effect on growth; if this was continued through two or more generations the effect became increasingly pronounced.

Adults

The calcium requirement of adults can be established by balance procedures on the assumption that the normal adult should be in zero calcium balance. It is a well established fact that normal individuals go into negative calcium balance at low calcium intakes and tend to go into positive calcium balance at high intakes. Somewhere between these extremes lies the intake at which the normal individual is in zero balance, *i.e.* the normal mean requirement. This mean normal calcium requirement was estimated by Mitchell and Curzon (1939) at about 500 mg and other estimates agree with this. We have now collected from the literature and analysed 212 calcium balances on 84 normal individuals and obtained a mean requirement of 500 mg/day. (The data were analysed by a quadratic function based on the known relation between calcium intake and calcium absorption of which we shall be publishing the details elsewhere.) The relationship between calcium intake and calcium output in these 212 normal balances can be seen in Fig. 1 which shows that the regression line meets the line of equality at 500 mg/day. This is the best estimate of calcium requirement in normal adults that we can obtain at the present time.

It is sometimes argued that short-term balances cannot provide an adequate measure of calcium requirement because of the phenomenon of 'adaptation' documented by Malm (1958) in his well-known study on male Norwegian prisoners. In this study he established after long periods on low calcium diets that the mean requirement of male adult prisoners (excluding certain cases that he regarded as osteoporotic) was 420 mg/day.

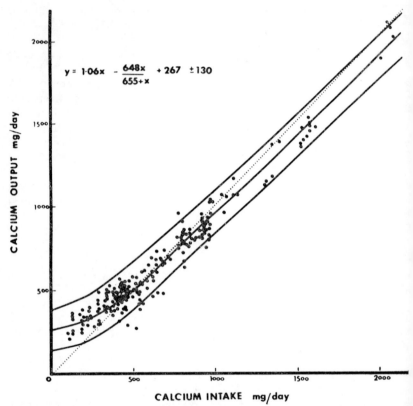

Fig. 1.   *Relation between calcium intake and calcium output in* 212 *calcium balances on* 84 *normal individuals. The dotted line indicates the line of equality.*

In absolute terms this figure is in fact only slightly lower than ours though on a bodyweight basis it is somewhat less because the average weight of his prisoners was greater than the average weight of our normal subjects. Nonetheless, these data are taken to signify that adaptation occurs and that the calcium intake of our society is too high. However, it is difficult to know what 'adaptation' really means. Normal individuals can of course 'adapt' to low calorie or low protein intakes by losing weight until a new plane of nutrition is established at which the nutrient intake is sufficient to maintain a constant bodyweight. This would hardly be taken, however, as a measure of the protein or energy requirement. Similarly, adaptation to a low calcium diet presumably takes place at the expense of the skeleton during the period of negative calcium balance before adaptation is established. In some of Malm's prisoners this period of adaptation took up to a year and represented a substantial calcium loss from the body. Whether it is wise or desirable or even scientifically sound to use such figures as the basis for calcium allowances seems extremely questionable.

Post-menopausal women

Women start to lose bone at the rate 1–2 %/annum when gonadal function declines in the fifth decade. This loss of bone can be measured on a plain hand radiograph (Barnett and Nordin, 1960). Post-menopausal loss of bone is associated with a steep rise in the incidence of lower forearm fractures and expresses itself in a slightly raised fasting plasma and urine calcium which can be restored to normal by the administration of oestrogens (Gallagher et al., 1972). This post-menopausal change in calcium metabolism appears to be due to an increase in the sensitivity of bone to parathyroid hormone in the absence of oestrogen (Nordin, 1971) and can probably be delayed if not entirely prevented by oestrogen replacement therapy (Meema and Meema, 1968).

Since calcium absorption does not change at the menopause (Bullamore et al., 1970) whereas urine calcium goes up, it could be argued that the post-menopausal state represents an increase in calcium requirement. To put it another way, the body's calcium economy is less efficient in the absence of oestrogens than it is when oestrogenic activity is normal. Many analogies to this situation can be found in other fields of endocrinology. For instance, the body's sodium economy is less efficient if aldosterone activity is reduced, but patients with Addison's disease can be maintained if the salt intake is high enough. Similarly the water economy is less efficient in the absence of antidiuretic hormone but patients with diabetes insipidus do survive if their water intake can be sufficiently increased. Thus the sodium requirement is increased in Addison's disease and the water requirement in diabetes insipidus. Similarly, we suggest the calcium requirement is increased in the absence of oestrogens.

There are not yet enough balance data in post-menopausal women to establish this point but the few balances which we have performed in this group have invariably shown a negative calcium balance on a calcium intake of about 500 mg attributable entirely to a relatively high urine calcium which can be reduced by oestrogen administration (Fig. 2). The question is whether this negative calcium balance due to a high urine calcium can be offset by the administration of calcium supplements, and

whether such calcium supplements would delay or prevent post-menopausal bone loss.

Preliminary results from a sequential study of hand X-rays in post-
menopausal women suggest that this may prove to be the case. As we have
reported elsewhere (Horsman and Nordin, 1973) metacarpal cortical area
can be measured on hand radiographs with needle calipers (Nordin and

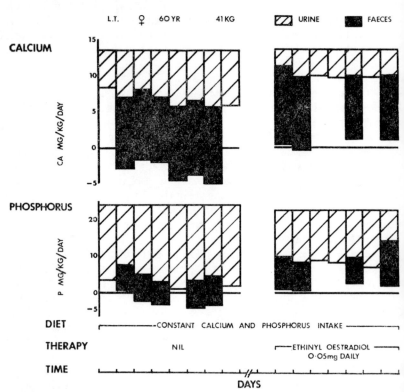

Fig. 2. Calcium and phosphorus balances in a post-menopausal woman before and on
ethinyloestradiol. There is a 3-month interval between the 3 balances. Note the fall in
urinary calcium and phosphorus with little change in calcium or phosphorus absorption.

Smith, 1965) with a measurement error as small as 0·1 mm. In serial
studies, the measurements are made in duplicate on six metacarpals.
Using this technique we have performed serial measurements on a series
of 43 post-menopausal women without overt bone disease for periods of
up to six years. Twenty-nine of these patients were on free diets, four on
low calcium diets and ten on calcium citrate supplements to provide an
additional gram of calcium daily. Figure 3 shows the relation between the

calcium intake (obtained by diet history) and cortical bone loss in these subjects. Within the normal range of dietary calcium intakes, there was no significant relation between dietary calcium and the rate of bone loss, but bone loss was clearly accelerated in the four subjects on low calcium diets and clearly reduced in the ten subjects on calcium supplements. These preliminary data, which we will be publishing in full elsewhere, suggest that post-menopausal osteoporosis is accelerated by a low calcium diet and retarded by a very high calcium intake and perhaps imply that the calcium allowance for post-menopausal women should be increased.

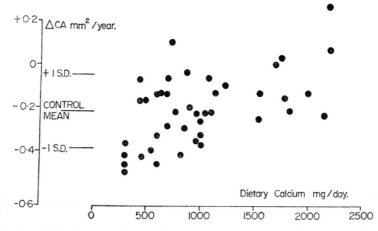

Fig. 3.   *Relation between dietary calcium and metacarpal cortical bone loss in 43 post-menopausal women. The 4 on the left were on low calcium diets. The 10 on the right were on calcium citrate supplements. The remainder on free diets.*

Old age

From the age of about 60–65 bone loss proceeds in both sexes until the end of life, and this is associated with a progressive rise in the femoral neck fracture rate, particularly in women in whom bone loss is more severe than in men. This phase is associated with a fall in calcium absorption which is also more pronounced in women than in men (Bullamore et al., 1970) and which is at least partially reversible with vitamin D (*see* below). Whether this decline in calcium absorption can be offset by increasing the calcium intake is not yet clear. If the malabsorption of calcium in old people is in fact due to vitamin D deficiency or an alteration in vitamin D metabolism then it is perhaps hardly correct to speak of an increase in calcium requirement when what in fact is happening is an increase in vitamin D requirement. It is therefore impossible to say at the present time what is the calcium requirement of old people.

VITAMIN D

Vitamin D requirement is more difficult to establish than calcium requirement because of the unknown contribution from ultraviolet irradiation of
the skin where 7-dehydrocholesterol is converted into cholecalciferol.
What is clear, however, is that rickets was relatively common in this
country—particularly in urban areas—until vitamin D was added to all
baby foods in 1944 in a concentration of 280 international units (iu)/ounce
of dried milk powder. Following an epidemic of infantile hypercalcaemia
this was reduced in 1957 to 115 iu/ounce which, together with the vitamin
drops now issued to babies, provide an infant with something like 500 iu
of vitamin D/day. This appears to be holding nutritional rickets at a
very low level except in immigrants who may not always be providing
their babies with the necessary supplements. The United Kingdom panel
on dietary allowances recommend 400 iu/day for children aged from 1 to
5 years and there seems no reason to question this recommendation at the
present time.

There is little evidence of vitamin D deficiency among young adults in
the United Kingdom other than those with absorptive defects, those on
anticonvulsant drugs (who have an altered vitamin D metabolism) and
some cases with other metabolic disorders, although nutritional osteomalacia is not uncommon in young immigrant women. This seems to
occur mainly in immigrants taking their native diet rather than those who
have adapted to the European diet but whether this is a critical factor or
whether it is the pigmentation of their skin, their protective clothing or
their diet which is the determining factor, is uncertain. Almost the only
significant source of vitamin D in the diet is margarine which is fortified
to the extent of about 300 iu/100 g. There is very little in natural dairy
products, and the amount varies with the time of year. The United Kingdom
panel recommends 100 iu daily for adults but they admit that very little
is known of the vitamin D requirement of adults.

The vitamin D requirement of the elderly is another matter. As has
already been indicated above, there is a progressive decline in calcium
absorption in both sexes after the age of about 60, more particularly in
women. In some subjects this malabsorption can be corrected with vitamin
D in a dose of 1000 iu daily but other cases may require 10 000 iu or even
more. It is thus impossible to say at the present time whether this represents
a true vitamin D deficiency in old people, whether there is malabsorption
of vitamin D or whether possibly there is some alteration in vitamin D
metabolism in the elderly which effectively increases their requirement. It
must be borne in mind that old people are frequently housebound, that
little or no ultraviolet light penetrates through glass windows and that the
diet of the elderly tends to be rather poor because appetite and income
decline with age.

Whether there is in fact a relative or absolute deficiency of vitamin D in old people, frequent reports of osteomalacia at this time of life (Chalmers *et al.*, 1967) strongly suggest that old people require additional vitamin D. In our experience, osteomalacia is present in at least 30% of cases of fractured neck of femur as judged by iliac crest biopsy, and we have been able to show (and will be reporting elsewhere) that this osteomalacia of old people responds to vitamin D therapy (Aaron, Gallagher and Nordin, in preparation). We are therefore inclined to the view that vitamin D supplementation is required at both extremes of life. Rickets has been largely abolished by giving vitamin D to babies. Is not the time approaching when osteomalacia in the elderly might be prevented by comparable supplementation to old people?

SUMMARY AND CONCLUSIONS

Much work remains to be done on the requirement of calcium and vitamin D before recommended allowances can rest on firm foundations. In the present state of knowledge the calcium allowances recommended by the United Kingdom panel appear too low for safety as far as children and post-menopausal women are concerned and the recommended vitamin D allowance may have to be increased substantially in old people if osteomalacia proves to be a significant factor in the pathogenesis of femoral neck fracture.

REFERENCES

Barnett, E. and Nordin, B. E. C. (1960). *Clin. Radiol.*, **11**, 166.

Bullamore, J. R., Gallagher, J. C., Wilkinson, R., Nordin, B. E. C. and Marsh, D. H. (1970). *Lancet*, **2**, 535.

Chalmers, J., Conacher, W. D. H., Gardner, D. L. and Scott, P. J. (1967). *J Bone Jt. Surg.*, **49B**, 403.

Gallagher, J. C., Young, M. M. and Nordin, B. E. C. (1972). *Clin. Endocr.*, **1**, 57.

Horsman, A. and Nordin, B. E. C. (1973). In *Proceedings of 9th European Symposium on Calcified Tissues, Vienna* 1972.

Jowsey, J. and Raisz, L. (1968). *Endocrinology*, **82**, 382.

Leitch, I. and Aitken, F. C. (1959). *Nutr. Abstr. Rev.*, **29**, 393.

Malm, O. J. (1958). *Calcium Requirement and Adaptation in Adult Men*, Oslo University Press, Oslo.

Meema, H. E. and Meema, S. (1968). *Can. med. Ass. J.*, **99**, 248.

Mitchell, H. H. and Curzon, E. G. (1939). *The Dietary Requirement of Calcium and its Significance*, Hermenn, Paris.

Nordin, B. E. C. (1960). *Clin. Orthop.*, **17**, 235.

Nordin, B. E. C. (1971). *Br. med. J.*, **1,** 571.
Nordin, B. E. C. (1973). In *Nutritional Deficiencies in Modern Society*, edited by
   A. N. Howard and I. McLean Baird, p. 27, Newman Books Ltd, London.
Nordin, B. E. C. and Smith, D. A. (1965). *Diagnostic Procedures in Disorders
   of Calcium Metabolism*, Churchill, London.
Rasmussen, H. and Arnaud, C. (1967). In *L'Osteomalacie*, edited by D. J. Hioco,
   p. 221, Masson, Paris.
Sherman, H. C. (1952). *Chemistry of Food and Nutrition*. Macmillan, New York.

CHAPTER 22

Nutritional needs of the elderly

A. N. EXTON-SMITH

Geriatric Department, University College Hospital, London

The Department of Health and Social Security (1972) has recently reported the results of a nutritional survey of the elderly population which was carried out in six centres, namely, Angus, Glasgow, Cambridge, the London Borough of Camden, Portsmouth and Sunderland. A diagnosis of malnutrition was made in 3 % of the elderly population surveyed and this included both protein–calorie malnutrition, iron deficiency and specific vitamin deficiencies. Rarely, however, was there a primary cause associated with social or economic factors and in the majority of cases an underlying medical condition was discovered to account for the malnutrition.

NUTRIENT INTAKES OF THE ELDERLY

Durnin (1964) recognised that the nutritional requirements may change owing to alteration in the amount of physical activity, to change in the weight or composition of the body and to decrease in muscular efficiency. He argues that these factors will cause little alteration in the body's gross metabolism and his and other studies show that the intake of nutrients and energy at the age of 60 or more seem similar to those at the age of 30 years. In the report 'Recommended Intakes of Nutrients for the United Kingdom' (Department of Health and Social Security, 1969) it is considered that although with increasing age there is a gradual decline in the metabolism at rest and therefore a reduced need for energy in the diet a relatively greater reduction results from a decline in physical activity of the individual. The recommendations for energy intakes for the elderly and the very old were based on judgment of the rates at which most people slow down in their activities. The recommended energy intakes assuming a sedentary life are 2350 kcal (9·8 MJ) for men aged 65 to 75 and 2100 kcal (8·8 MJ) for men aged 75 and over; for women aged 55 to 75 and for those 75 and over the corresponding recommended intakes are 2050 kcal (8·6 MJ) and 1900 kcal (8·0 MJ) respectively. The report, however, emphasises that there are many old people who retain their active habits of life until they are 75 or over and that they need more energy in their diet than the figures indicated above. Thus it is clearly necessary when making recommendations for the nutrient intakes of older people based on results of nutrition surveys to include a medical examination of the subjects in order to distinguish those who are fit and active from those who suffer from a decline in their activities due to some underlying medical disorder (Exton-Smith, 1970). The need for making this distinction is all the more striking in advanced old age when the proportion of the population with physical and mental disabilities increases considerably. There have been a number of recent studies which have been made to assess the nutritional needs of the elderly and to investigate the relationship between nutrition and health.

THE OCCURRENCE OF NUTRITIONAL DEFICIENCIES

Although the individual dietary pattern in the majority of old people remains similar to that which has been acquired by habits developed at a younger age there are many factors which begin to operate more often with increasing age and these may lead to marked alterations in nutritional intake. Some of these factors are related to decline in bodily health and difficulty in obtaining and preparing food, to the changed circumstances which follow retirement, and to social isolation, loneliness following bereavement and ignorance of what constitutes a balanced diet, especially in the widower who must cater for himself for the first time. The primary and secondary causes of malnutrition are summarised in Table 1 and their importance has been discussed elsewhere (Exton-Smith, 1963).

TABLE 1

PRIMARY AND SECONDARY CAUSES OF
MALNUTRITION

Primary	Secondary
Ignorance	Impaired appetite
Loneliness	Inefficient mastication
Physical disability	Intestinal malabsorption
Mental disorder	Alcoholism
Iatrogenic	Drugs
Poverty	Increased requirements

These are the common causes, but it must be remembered that malnutrition at this age is often multifactorial in origin. Some of the deficiencies which occur are described below.

Vitamin B complex
A high incidence of changes in the mucous membranes of the tongue and lips associated with B complex deficiency has been reported by Griffiths

et al. (1967) and by Brocklehurst *et al.* (1968). The classical sign of nicotinic acid deficiency is a raw 'beef-red' tongue and riboflavin deficiency leads to angular stomatitis, magenta tongue and seborrhoea of the naso-labial folds. But some of these changes can also occur in iron deficiency and vitamin B_{12} deficiency, following the administration of broad spectrum antibiotics and as a result of oral infection with *Candida albicans*. The commonest cause of angular stomatitis in the elderly is the ill-fitting of dentures.

There is conflict of opinion on the extent to which abnormal tongue signs can be corrected. Dymock and Brocklehurst (1972) repeated their earlier studies and used single vitamin supplementation instead of a multivitamin preparation on 77 old people in hospital who survived for the one year's clinical trial. Riboflavin therapy was associated with a significant improvement in cheilosis and nicotinamide produced an improvement in the dorsum of the tongue. MacLeod (1972), on the other hand, failed to confirm these findings. In a series of 80 patients with abnormal tongue appearance vitamin supplementation for one year had no effect on the tongue changes or the signs of angular stomatitis. Similar negative results were obtained in the series investigated by Berry and Darke (1972). Thus of the 27 patients who had lesions of the lip or angle of the mouth 24 did not improve after one year's administration of a riboflavin containing tablet. Moreover, in the 66 elderly patients who had abnormal appearances of the dorsum of the tongue there was no statistical difference in the response rate between those who received vitamin B supplementation and those who were treated with a placebo tablet. In 90 % of the subjects who had changes in the dorsal surface of the tongue a fungal infection was found and Berry and Darke consider that this is the most likely cause of these changes.

In the nutrition study sponsored by the Department of Health and Social Security (1972), a special attempt was made to relate changes in mucous membranes to riboflavin deficiency. Of the 778 subjects examined 57 were diagnosed as having either angular stomatitis or cheilosis. The mean intake of riboflavin for those subjects with these lip lesions was 1·2 mg/day compared with a mean intake of 1·3 mg/day for those without lip lesions; these differences are not statistically significant. Out of the 23 subjects who had very low intakes of riboflavin (less than 0·7 mg for males and 0·55 mg for females) four subjects had lip lesions. Thus, although there may be some element of clinical ariboflavinosis in the elderly population, the numbers must be very small and in general the riboflavin status appeared to be satisfactory. It is apparent that there is a discrepancy between the clinical findings and the expectation based on low dietary intakes of riboflavin.

In the study of accidental hypothermia in the elderly conducted in a random sample of the elderly population of Camden (Fox *et al.*, 1973) a limited investigation of the nutritional status of the subjects was made. In 128 subjects who attended hospital for clinical examination and other tests Thurnham (1972) measured the erythrocyte glutathione reductase activity (EGR) and the percentage stimulation of EGR by flavin adenine dinucleotide (FAD). A stimulation of greater than 30 % was found in 18 % of the males and in 19 % of the females. Thus it is considered that there may be marginal riboflavin deficiency in about one-fifth of the elderly population. However, the true clinical significance of low riboflavin levels (and of other vitamins) is at present not known.

A similar uncertainty exists about the exact levels of folic acid in the serum or red cells which are considered to be adequate. Herbert (1967) maintains that folic acid deficiency is the commonest vitamin deficiency in man. Although a folate-free diet quickly leads to lowering of the serum folate levels, many months elapse before clinical or haematological changes develop. In a survey of elderly patients admitted to the Geriatric Department of a London Hospital, Hurdle and Williams (1966) found serum folate levels of less than 5 ng/ml in 39 % of consecutive admissions. Read *et al.* (1965) in Bristol found that 80 % of fifty entrants to old people's homes had folate deficiency, which they took as a level of less than 6 ng/ml. Such lower limits, however, do not represent very strict criteria of deficiency. Batata *et al.* (1967) in Oxford adopted a lower limit of normal of 2·1 ng/ml and found that 10 % of patients over the age of 60 admitted to hospital had levels below this limit. A nutritional origin was suspected since with severe physical disability (and in consequence inability of the patient to look after himself) the more likely was there to be folate deficiency; there was found to be a statistically significant correlation between organic brain disease and low folate levels.

In the Nutrition Survey of the Elderly (Department of Health and Social Security, 1972) 15 % of the subjects had serum folate levels of less than 3 ng/ml and 3·7 % of the subjects had red cell folate levels of less than 100 ng/ml. There was no apparent relationship between haemoglobin concentration and the serum and red cell folate levels. Of the 22 subjects with low red cell folate from the 629 people in whom haemoglobin and red cell folates were measured only two women were mildly anaemic. In this study there was no significant relationship between folate levels or the clinicians' assessment of mental state.

Vitamin C
Although scurvy is now a rare disease, occasional cases are found amongst the elderly especially in men. The manifestations include weakness, anaemia, swelling and bleeding of the gums, 'sheet' haemorrhages in the skin of the arms and legs, and sometimes haemorrhages at other sites. Sublingual 'petechiae' have been regarded as an early sign of vitamin C deficiency, but Andrews *et al.* (1969) have shown by histological examination that these

lesions are usually not haemorrhages but small aneurysmal dilatations of the minute vessels under the tongue. They do not disappear when the vitamin C intake is increased and it is unlikely therefore that they are due to acute vitamin C deficiency.

It seems likely that the bodily stores of vitamin C in many old people are diminished and low levels of leucocyte ascorbic acid have been reported by several observers; the levels are lower in the elderly than in younger subjects (Brook and Grimshaw, 1968), lower in winter than in summer (Andrews et al., 1966), and lower in men than in women (Allen et al., 1967). In a recent study Milne et al. (1971) in Edinburgh measured the leucocyte ascorbic acid (LAA) levels and the vitamin C intakes in a random sample of 204 men and 247 women; the mean levels for women $(23{\cdot}88 \ \mu g/10^8$ white blood corpuscles) were found to be significantly higher than for men $(18{\cdot}11 \ \mu g/10^8$ wbc). The values decreased with increasing age in women but not in men. They were significantly higher in both sexes in the six months July to December. Fifty per cent of men and 58% of women had intakes of less than 30 mg daily, 23·6% of men and 28·1% of women had intakes of less than 20 mg daily and 4·7% of men and 3% of women intakes less than 10 mg daily. A significantly greater proportion of both men and women had mean intakes of less than 30 mg daily in the months October to March compared with the months April to September. A moderate correlation was present between vitamin C intake and LAA level. It was also found that LAA levels increase in parallel with but lag behind seasonal increases in vitamin C intakes.

The Edinburgh study and other dietary surveys disclose that there is an appreciable number of old people who have an intake of less than 10 mg daily which is known to be the amount required to prevent or cure scurvy (Bartley et al., 1953). A high proportion of the elderly population are consuming less than the recommended allowance of 30 mg/day (Department of Health and Social Security, 1969); this allowance takes into account the changes in requirements due to stress and the considerable individual variations in requirements which are known to exist (Srikantia et al., 1970). The majority of people will not suffer from any ill effects with a vitamin C intake of less than 30 mg, but our assessment is handicapped through a lack of information of the levels of LAA required for the maintenance of health. Windsor and Williams (1970) have attempted to determine the significance of low LAA levels by measuring the total hydroxyproline excretion (THP) in the urine of elderly subjects with differing vitamin C status. THP is a measure of collagen metabolism and vitamin C is required for collagen synthesis. It was found that in old people with LAA levels of less than $15 \ \mu g/10^8$ wbc the administration of vitamin C produced a rise in THP excretion whereas this did not occur when the LAA content was greater than $15 \ \mu g/10^8$ wbc. It is reasonable to suppose that subclinical or clinical deficiency exists in people with LAA levels of less than 15 μg/10^8 wbc and there is evidence from studies in which this parameter has been measured that levels below this lower limit are commonly found in old people.

Thus Thurnham (1972) in an investigation of the old people who partici-pated in the Camden Survey of accidental hypothermia found that 28% of the men and 10% of the women had LAA levels equal to or less than 15 μg/10^8 wbc. The much higher proportion of men with low levels is in keeping with the findings of the Edinburgh and other surveys and accords with clinical experience that men are more prone to scurvy than women.

Wilson *et al.* (1972) in Cornwall have reported the relationship between LAA levels and mortality in the aged. Determination of LAA was made on 159 patients admitted to a geriatric department. It was found that the mortality within the first four weeks in hospital was 47% for those whose LAA level on admission was less than 12 μg/10^8 wbc, compared with 10% when the initial LAA was greater than 25 μg/10^8 wbc (p < 0.01). This significant difference in mortality between the high and low LAA groups might be related to severity of illness or special clinical features. Wilson *et al.* (1972) found no marked difference in clinical features (the incidence of such conditions as cerebrovascular disease, congestive heart failure and malignant disease being similar in the two groups), but the overall severity of the illness appeared to be greater in the group with low LAA levels. Thus from this study it was not possible to say whether the vitamin C status influenced mortality directly or whether the severity of illness affected both the nutritional status and mortality. It is believed that low LAA levels can be raised by the administration of vitamin C, but whether this occurs in patients who are severely ill is uncertain. Nor is it known what benefit is derived from an elevation of tissue vitamin C levels.

Vitamin D

Deficiency of vitamin D may result from several factors and those which are most commonly found in old age include: inadequate dietary intake, lack of exposure to sunlight, intestinal malabsorption and renal disease. Sometimes these causes occur together, for example, mild degrees of mal-absorption in an old person who is housebound and having a low dietary intake.

The occurrence of vitamin D deficiency due to low dietary intake was assessed in the first King Edward's Hospital Fund survey (Exton-Smith and Stanton, 1965). Following the dietary investigations three-quarters of the elderly women agreed to participate in further studies involving clinical assessment, biochemical investigations and the determination of the radio-graphic density of bone (Exton-Smith *et al.*, 1966). Slightly more than a quarter of the subjects were found to have marked skeletal rarefaction and when these subjects were compared with age-matched individuals whose bones were of higher density it was found that the former had significantly lower vitamin D intakes. Moreover, vitamin D intakes were correlated with alterations in the serum levels of calcium, inorganic phosphorus and alkaline phosphatase. Thus the findings of this study suggest that dietary vitamin D deficiency may contribute to the skeletal rarefaction which is so common in old age.

Smith *et al.* (1964) in the United States assessed the vitamin D status of a group of women living in Michigan (average age 60·6 years) and compared them with a group of women of similar age living in Puerto Rico. For the Michigan group the level of vitamin D in the blood (serum antirachitic activity) was significantly lower in those subjects with low bone density compared with those having normal bones and the level showed marked seasonal variation. By contrast, in Puerto Rico, where there is much greater exposure to sunlight and a higher vitamin D content of the food, the incidence of skeletal rarefaction was much lower, the serum vitamin D levels were much higher and there was no seasonal variation. The authors attributed the skeletal rarefaction to osteoporosis, rather than to osteomalacia, but they noted a correlation between the vitamin D levels and the serum calcium, inorganic phosphorus and alkaline phosphatase.

Clinical osteomalacia may not be rare in certain sections of the elderly population. Thus Anderson *et al.* (1966) in Glasgow found 16 cases after thorough investigation of 100 women admitted to a geriatric department and who had a possible clinical indication, namely, vague and generalised pain, bone tenderness, low backache, muscle weakness and stiffness, waddling gait, skeletal deformity, malabsorption states, long confinement indoors or malnutrition. Subsequently 100 admissions to the female geriatric wards were investigated and the incidence of osteomalacia was found to be 4% of all elderly women.

The importance of detecting osteomalacia lies in the fact that the condition is so readily preventable by increased vitamin D intake and the disease when it is recognised responds most satisfactorily to simple treatment. Particular attention must be paid to the housebound who probably represent the largest single vulnerable group. The recent study of housebound old people (Exton-Smith *et al.*, 1972) has disclosed that 48% of housebound women aged 70 to 79 years have a vitamin D intake of less than 30 iu/day compared with 13% of active women of similar age. For those confined to the house lack of exposure to sunlight is a significant additional factor.

Chalmers *et al.* (1967) have recognised the importance of vitamin D deficiency in the causation of fractures and other orthopaedic problems in the elderly. They describe the clinical features of 37 patients with osteomalacia and they emphasise the need for thorough screening of all elderly patients, especially women, who present with weakness, skeletal pain, pathological fractures or diminished radiographic density of bone. Nordin (1971) has suggested that the majority of cases of vitamin D deficiency are recognised only at an advanced stage when the typical biochemical findings or bone changes of osteomalacia have developed, but long continued mild deficiency may also be responsible for osteoporosis. This he attributes to the vitamin D lack causing further impairment of calcium absorption which is already reduced in old age.

IMPROVING NUTRITION

The First Report of the Panel on the Nutrition of the Elderly (Department of Health and Social Security, 1970) stated that 'there is little doubt that more is known of the nutritional state of our nation than of any other in the world, but in relation to the elderly the evidence is still inadequate'. In old people it is often difficult to distinguish between the effects of nutritional factors which are operating for the first time in old age and those which may have influenced nutritional status many years previously and even in childhood. This difficulty is clearly seen in relation to the problem of bone rarefaction in old age. There is considerable evidence that the liability to osteoporosis in the elderly is determined at least in part by the skeletal development before maturity. Since child nutrition is better today than it was half a century ago, it is possible that the present generation of young people when they reach old age will suffer from less osteoporosis than is found in old people now.

In most forms of nutritional deficiency in the elderly, however, the factors responsible can be defined. But malnutrition when found rarely results from social and environmental causes alone and is often multi-factorial in origin.

Vulnerable groups
Old people especially at risk are the recently bereaved, the socially isolated (especially those with impairment of the special senses), those with mental disorders, very old people, and those who have not consulted their general practitioners for six months or more. Unless these vulnerable groups of old people can be recognised preventive measures would have to be applied to all old people irrespective of the fact that the majority will never suffer from nutritional deficiencies. The inefficiency and the undesirability of employing such procedures can only be overcome by identification of those especially at risk. The application of preventive measures to these smaller groups rather than to the whole elderly population becomes a manageable proposition.

We now believe that the housebound form the largest single group at risk. As a result of a recent investigation of the dietary and state of health of housebound old people (Exton-Smith et al., 1972) it has been shown that their vitamin C and vitamin D intakes (as well as the intakes of other nutrients) are substantially lower than those of active old people of comparable age. Physical and mental disability in old age not only affect the mode of living of those afflicted but also lead to alterations in their dietary pattern and nutritional status. The prevention of malnutrition in this group should present less difficulty than for other vulnerable groups of old people who cannot be so readily identified since the majority of the housebound are known to the health and social services.

General measures

Having identified the groups of old people especially at risk the individual's nutritional status must be assessed and if a dietary insufficiency is found means must be sought for improving his nutrient intake. The assessment of dietary intakes should ideally be made by dietitians, but their skills are rarely available for old people at home. Simple scoring systems have been devised (Marr *et al.*, 1961) and these are usually based on the number of main meals and the frequency of consumption of certain foods containing protein (meat, cheese, eggs, bread and milk). Such a system can be readily applied by a health visitor to give a rough guide on the quality of the diet. Ignorance about food and of what constitutes a balanced diet is very common amongst the elderly, especially widowers, and to remedy this instruction must be given by dietitians or health visitors.

Possible means of improving the nutrient intake of old people at home have been discussed elsewhere (Exton-Smith, 1968). They include encouraging those old people who are able to do so to eat at a club in the company of others and for less active (especially the housebound) the provision of an efficient meals on wheels service at least five days per week. The destruction of a considerable amount of vitamin C during the preparation of these meals must be borne in mind (Exton-Smith and Stanton, 1965) and this occurs to a greater degree than in meals prepared at home. The recipients of meals on wheels tend to regard the meal as the main one of the day; the meals must therefore be as nutritious as possible.

Supplementation

The most satisfactory means of improving nutrition is by improving the quality, and in some instances, the quantity of the diet. The very low intakes of certain vitamins, notably vitamins C and D must lead to consideration of the possibility of supplementation. Thus for those whose consumption of vitamin C is inadequate intake should be improved by the addition to the diet of citrus fruit, blackcurrant juice, rose hip syrup or tomatoes.

The alternative method of increasing intake by the prescription of vitamin C tablets is satisfactory but less desirable. Similar considerations apply to riboflavin and to folic acid but the extent to which the subjects would benefit from raising the serum or tissue levels of these vitamins is doubtful.

There is known to be considerable individual variation in requirements for vitamin D and since in some persons moderately excessive intakes can lead to vitamin D intoxication widespread supplementation could be harmful. A means of increasing the intake would be by the fortification of milk which is a procedure adopted in the United States, but the distribution of fortified milk would best be restricted to housebound old people for whom the intake of vitamin D is often low and its synthesis in the skin is inadequate through lack of exposure to sunlight.

The policy of introducing supplementation should only be decided after the results of carefully controlled experiments are available to assess the benefits of increased intakes. Once the practice of supplementation has become widespread it is difficult to prove or assess the benefits. Moreover, there is an understandable reluctance to withdraw a prophylactic measure on the basis of doubts about its value when it has been practised for several years.

REFERENCES

Allen, M. A., Andrews, J. and Brook, M. (1967). *Nutrition, Lond.*, **21,** 136.

Anderson, I., Campbell, A. E. R., Dunn, A. and Runciman, J. B. M. (1966). *Scott. med. J.*, **11,** 429.

Andrews, J., Brook, M. and Allen, M. A. (1966). *Geront. Clin. (Basel),* **8,** 257.

Andrews, J., Letcher, M. and Brook, M. (1969). *Br. med. J.*, **2,** 416.

Bartley, W., Krebs, H. A. and O'Brien, J. R. P. (1953). *Vitamin C Requirements of Human Adults,* Spec. Rep. Ser. med. Res. Coun. No. 280, HMSO, London.

Batata, M., Spray, G. H., Bolton, F. G., Higgins, G. and Wollner, L. (1967). *Br. med. J.*, **2,** 667.

Berry, W. T. C. and Darke, S. J. (1972). *Age and Ageing,* **1,** 177.

Brocklehurst, J., Griffiths, L. L., Taylor, G. F., Marks, J. and Scott, D. L. (1968). *Geront. Clin. (Basel),* **10,** 309.

Brook, M. and Grimshaw, J. J. (1968). *Am. J. clin. Nutr.*, **21,** 1254.

Chalmers, J., Conacher, W. D. H., Gardner, D. L. and Scott, P. J. (1967). *J. Bone Jt Surg.*, **49B,** 403.

Department of Health and Social Security (1969). *Recommended Intakes of Nutrients for the United Kingdom,* Rep pub. Hlth and med. Subj., No. 120, HMSO, London.

Department of Health and Social Security (1970). *First Report of the Panel on the Nutrition of the Elderly,* Rep. pub. Hlth and med. Subj., No. 123, HMSO, London.

Department of Health and Social Security (1972). *A Nutrition Survey of the Elderly,* Rep. Hlth and soc. Subj., No. 3, HMSO, London.

Durnin, J. V. G. A. (1964). In *Current Achievements in Geriatrics*, edited by
    W. F. Anderson and N. Isaacs, Cassell, London.
Dymock, S. and Brocklehurst, J. (1972). Paper given at Meeting of British
    Geriatrics Society, London.
Exton-Smith, A. N. (1963). *Nutrition, Lond.*, **17**, 5.
Exton-Smith, A. N. (1968). *R. Soc. Hlth J.*, **88**, 205.
Exton-Smith, A. N. (1970). *Nutrition, Lond.*, **24**, 218.
Exton-Smith, A. N. and Stanton, B. R. (1965). *An Investigation of the Dietary
    of Elderly Women Living Alone*, King Edward's Hospital Fund, London.
Exton-Smith, A. N., Hodkinson, H. M. and Stanton, B. R. (1966). *Lancet*, **2**,
    999.
Exton-Smith, A. N., Stanton, B. R. and Windsor, A. C. M. (1972). *Nutrition of
    Housebound Old People*, King Edward's Hospital Fund, London.
Fox, R. H., Woodward, P. M., Exton-Smith, A. N., Green, M. F., Donnison,
    D. V. and Wicks, M. H. (1973). *Br. med. J.*, **1**, 200.
Griffiths, L. L., Brocklehurst, J. C., Scott, D. L., Marks, J. and Blackley, J.
    (1967). *Geront. Clin. (Basel)*, **9**, 1.
Herbert, V., (1967). *Am. J. clin. Nutr.*, **20**, 562.
Hurdle, A. D. F. and Williams, T. C. P. (1966). *Br. med. J.*, **2**, 202.
MacLeod, R. D. (1972). *Age and Ageing*, **1**, 99.
Marr, J., Heady, J. A. and Morris, J. (1961). In *Proc. 3rd Int. Congress Dietetics*,
    p. 85, Newman Books Ltd, London.
Milne, J. S., Lonergen, M. E., Williamson, J., Moore, F. M. L., McMaster, R.
    and Percy, N. (1971). *Br. med. J.*, **4**, 383.
Nordin, B. E. C. (1971). *Br. med. J.*, **1**, 571.
Read, A. E., Gough, K. R., Pardoe, J. L. and Nicholas, A. (1965). *Br. med. J.*,
    2, 843.
Smith, R. W., Rizek, J., Frame, B. and Mansour, J. (1964). *Am. J. clin. Nutr.*,
    14, 98.
Srikantia, S. G., Mohanram, M. and Krishnaswamy, K. (1970). *Am. J. clin.
    Nutr.*, **23**, 59.
Thurnham, D. (1972). Personal communication.
Wilson, T. S., Weeks, M. M., Mukherjee, S. K., Murrell, J. S. and Andrews,
    C. T. (1972). *Geront. clin. (Basel)*, **14**, 17.
Windsor, A. C. M. and Williams, C. B. (1970). *Br. med. J.*, **1**, 731.

CHAPTER 23

1α-Hydroxycholecalciferol as a substitute for the kidney hormone, 1,25-dihydroxycholecalciferol, in an anephric patient

E. KODICEK

Director, Dunn Nutritional Laboratory, Cambridge

The interesting papers by Professor Nordin and Dr Exton-Smith (this volume) raise the question whether the requirement for vitamin D is not increased in old age. However, it is more likely that the appearance of vitamin D deficiency in the elderly is associated with an impairment of the intermediary metabolism of the vitamin.

It is now established that the vitamin D molecule undergoes certain changes in the body before it is converted to the active metabolite. This entails a hydroxylation at carbon 25 by the liver to form 25-hydroxychole-calciferol (Blunt *et al.*, 1968). This substance is then transported to the kidney where a hydroxyl function is inserted at carbon 1 to result in 1,25-dihydroxycholecalciferol, which has been called the kidney hormone (Fraser and Kodicek, 1970; Lawson *et al.*, 1971; Holick *et al.*, 1971).

In chronic renal failure, the impairment of the hydroxylation mechanism results in lack of formation of the kidney hormone, with a consequential lowering of intestinal calcium absorption and development of osteo-dystrophy (Mawer *et al.*, 1973).

To bypass the kidney hydroxylation mechanism, Dr Pelc in my laboratory has synthesised an analogue of vitamin D which contains a hydroxyl group at carbon 1 in α-position, namely 1α-hydroxycholecalciferol (1α-OHCC) (Fig. 1). The substance has the same antirachitic activity as vitamin D_3; it has, in the chicken, a positive effect on Ca transport from gut and on Ca mobilisation from the bones (Cruickshank *et al.*, 1973).

It is at present uncertain whether these effects by the 1α-OHCC are dependent on a further hydroxylation at C 25 by liver to form 1,25-di-hydroxycholecalciferol; nevertheless it appears to be a possible therapeutic agent in chronic renal failure.

I wish to report a case of a patient without kidneys, suffering from osteodystrophy and hyperparathyroidism, to whom 1α-hydroxycholecal-ciferol was administered. This treatment was done in collaboration with Drs T. M. Chalmers, J. O. Hunter, M. W. Davie and K. F. Szaz, of

Addenbrooke's Hospital, Cambridge. The 37-year-old patient had been uraemic for 2 years with chronic sclerosing glomerulonephritis. Bilateral nephrectomy was performed 2 months ago and he had been maintained by intermittent dialysis. Skeletal X-rays revealed severe osteodystrophy in the spine, skull, clavicles and extremities. Bone biopsy showed increased osteoblastic and osteoclastic activity and wide osteoid seams.

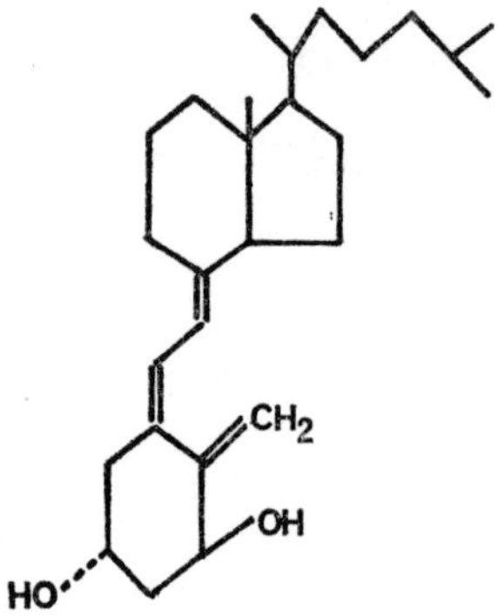

1α-HO-5,6-cis CHOLECALCIFEROL

Figure 1

As can be seen from Table 1, 6 doses of the order of 2·5 μg produced only a slight response; however, an increase to 30 μg for 3 days resulted in a doubling of the calcium absorption rate and in a significant rise in serum calcium, which did not exceed normality. It should be noted that the serum calcium returned to pre-dosing levels 8 days after the last

TABLE 1

RECORD OF TESTS FOR CALCIUM ABSORPTION AND SERUM CALCIUM BEFORE AND AFTER TREATMENT WITH 1α-HYDROXYCHOLECALCIFEROL OF AN ANEPHRIC PATIENT

Day	*Treatment*	Ca^{47} *absorption*[a] (%)	*Serum calcium* (*mg/100 ml*)
1	None	33 ± 2	9·3
5–11	$6 \times 2·5$ μg 1α-OHCC, i.v.	—	9·5–9·8
13	—	41 ± 3	9·6
23–25	3×30 μg 1α-OHCC, i.v.	—	10·2
26	—	69 ± 4	10·4
33	—	—	9·7

[a] Four-hour fractional Ca^{47} absorption by the arm-counting technique of Pak *et al*. (1972).

injection of 1α-OHCC. We believe that we have been able to substitute for the missing kidney activity by the vitamin D analogue. This treatment is being repeated in other patients. It is hoped that 1α-OHCC will prove less toxic than 1,25-dihydroxycholecalciferol, which caused severe hypercalcaemia when administered (Brickman *et al.*, 1972).

ACKNOWLEDGEMENTS

We are grateful to Professor R. Y. Calne and Dr D. B. Evans for giving us the opportunity to study the patient, and to Dr D. P. D. Wight for reporting on the bone biopsy.

REFERENCES

Blunt, J. W., DeLuca, H. F. and Schnoes, H. K. (1968)., *Biochemistry, N.Y.*, **7**, 3317.
Brickman, A. S., Coburn, J. W. and Norman, A. W. (1972). *New Engl. J. Med.*, **287**, 891.
Cruickshank, E. M., Lawson, D. E. M. and Kodicek, E. (1973). Unpublished data.
Fraser, D. R. and Kodicek, E. (1970). *Nature, Lond.*, **228**, 764.
Holick, M. F., Schnoes, H. K. and DeLuca, H. F. (1971). *Proc. natn. Acad. Sci. USA*, **68**, 803.
Lawson, D. E. M., Fraser, D. R., Kodicek, E., Morris, H. R. and Williams, D. H. (1971). *Nature, Lond.*, **230**, 228.
Mawer, E. B., Backhouse, J., Taylor, C. M., Lumb, Q. A. and Stanbury, S. W. (1973). *Lancet*, **1**, 626.
Pak, C. Y. C., East, D. A., Sanzenbacher, L. J., Delea, C. S. and Bartter, F. C. (1972). *J. clin. Endocr. Metab.*, **35**, 261.

PART 5

IMPLICATIONS OF MODERN NUTRITIONAL
THOUGHT FOR THE FOOD INDUSTRY

CHAPTER 24

The changing composition of food

A. W. HUBBARD

Department of Trade and Industry,
Laboratory of the Government Chemist, London

In recent years intensive farming practices and new food processing techniques have attracted a great deal of public attention; and some concern has been expressed about the nutritive value of such products in comparison with those obtained by traditional or conventional means. Some beef cattle are now raised intensively on diets containing a considerable amount of barley; a large proportion of chickens and eggs available in retail trade are produced intensively in battery or deep litter units; and a considerable amount of the most popular type of bread eaten in Britain is now made by a process which involves intense mechanical agitation of the dough in special high speed mixers. Affluence, world travel and the increase in leisure time has led to an increasing interest in convenience foods, exotic foods, snacks, slimming foods and dishes suitable for informal dining. To meet the demands the food industry imports foods from all parts of the world, produces more sophisticated products and makes greater use of food additives to prevent or retard deterioration and to provide a wider choice of foods of uniform quality available throughout the year. Foods are tailored for specific use, for example, slimming foods and foods for special dietary use. The increasing use of food additives, pesticides and artificial fertilisers coupled with environmental pollution has resulted in a further class of food namely the 'health' and 'natural' foods.

These are matters of importance to several Government departments with an interest in the nutritional quality of food. Therefore, in 1965 the Ministry of Agriculture, Fisheries and Food formed a Committee on Food Composition to coordinate the investigational work done by Government departments on food composition; to consider the need for further work; and to disseminate the results of collaborative studies. The Committee includes representatives of the Ministry of Agriculture, Fisheries and Food, the Department of Health and Social Security, the Ministry of Defence, the Department of Education and Science, the Agricultural and Medical Research Councils and the Laboratory of the Government Chemist. Several of the studies initiated by this Committee have been published (Robertson *et al.*, 1966; Chamberlain *et al.*, 1966; Harries *et al.*,

1968), and in these papers the nutritive value of broiler chickens, Chorley-wood process bread and barley beef has been compared with that of these commodities produced by traditional methods of husbandry or processing. It is the aim of this paper to survey these collaborative studies and to outline the results of more recent work on eggs, bread and potatoes which has been carried out in the Laboratory of the Government Chemist on behalf of the Committee, and, in addition, to consider newer developments which have led to changes in the composition of food which may have nutritional significance.

BROILER AND FREE RANGE CHICKENS

One of the main objectives of the study by Robertson et al. (1966) was to compare the composition of the raw and cooked meat of broiler and free range chickens. In a pilot study six broiler chickens processed commercially for retail sale were compared with six free range cockerels prepared by a family butcher, results being obtained for moisture, protein, fat and thiamin on both raw and cooked meat. This exercise was followed by the

TABLE 1

MOISTURE, PROTEIN, FAT AND THIAMIN CONTENT OF TOTAL CHICKEN MEAT PER 100 g EDIBLE PORTION (FLESH ONLY)

Type of chicken	Preparation	Moisture (g)	Protein (g)	Fat (g)	Thiamin (µg)
PILOT STUDY					
Frozen broiler	Raw	74·2	21·7	4·2	60
	Cooked	68·0	25·1	6·0	39
Fresh free range	Raw	72·8	22·0	3·3	97
	Cooked	68·5	25·5	4·9	66
MAIN STUDY					
Fresh broiler	Raw	74·5	21·0	3·44	41
	Cooked	66·2	28·5	6·14	27
Frozen broiler	Raw	74·2	23·8	3·45	36
	Cooked	64·8	28·9	6·10	25
Fresh free range (Sykes Hybrid 3)	Raw	75·0	21·9	1·60	60
	Cooked	66·9	30·4	2·89	49
Fresh free range (Light Sussex × Rhode Island Red)	Raw	72·7	24·1	4·74	46
	Cooked	65·5	29·4	6·13	34

Reference: Robertson et al. (1966).

main study in which 48 oven-ready birds supplied by the research station of a large company were used in the comparison of 12 fresh and 12 frozen broiler chickens with 12 small free range Sykes hybrid 3 cockerels and 12 slightly heavier free range cockerels (Light Sussex × Rhode Island Red). In addition to estimates of the yield of meat, the edible portion of fresh and frozen broiler chicken and the losses on cooking, results were obtained for the moisture, protein, fat and thiamin contents of white meat from the breast and red meat from the legs, wings and backs. A summary of the results for both the pilot and main studies is given in Table 1 which is taken from Robertson *et al.* (1966). The results show that there is little difference between the moisture and protein contents of the meat of the broiler and free range chickens. Some differences were found in the fat content which appeared to be related to breed as well as the type of bird rather than to age or weight. In both the pilot and main studies the flesh of the free range chickens contained more thiamin than the broiler meat but this is of no nutritional significance in a mixed diet since, in the average household diet, poultry supplies less than 1% of the total thiamin.

BREAD

Since the Chorleywood bread process (CBP) for making bread was introduced in 1961 by the Flour Milling and Baking Research Association it has rapidly replaced the conventional methods of bread production so that over 75% of all bread baked in Britain is now produced by this process. One of the main features of the new technique is that the bulk fermentation of the dough for periods of 2 to 4 hours is replaced by a few minutes of intense mechanical agitation in special mixers. Other features of the process include the use of ascorbic acid as an improver, the addition of extra water and yeast and the use of softer wheats. The general quality of the bread produced is superior in most instances to that made by conventional methods and the process has the advantages that overall production time is reduced from 5 hours to $1\frac{3}{4}$ hours, the yield of bread is increased and there is a considerable saving in factory space. To determine whether the nutrient content of the bread produced by the new process differed in any major respect from conventional bread, loaves were made at a commercial bakery by both methods using a weak and a strong flour. Some bread was also made in a pilot scale bakery for tests on net protein utilisation values. Both the bread and the flours were examined for moisture, protein, fat, ash, thiamin, nicotinic acid, ascorbic acid and net protein utilisation values from which it was concluded that bread made by the Chorleywood bread process is indistinguishable from conventional bread except for slightly higher values for moisture and thiamin. No ascorbic or dehydroascorbic acid was detected in the bread. Details of the study are given by Chamberlain *et al.* (1966). Although the results of the study suggest that the difference in nutrient content of the two types of bread is small it was thought desirable to examine in greater detail samples of CBP and conventionally made loaves purchased at retail outlets throughout Britain. Some 70 large, sliced, wrapped loaves of CBP bread and 64 conventionally made loaves were obtained at shops throughout Britain over a period of 10 months by staff of the Flour Milling and Baking Research Association. After determining the moisture content at the laboratories of the Research Association the samples were sent to the Laboratory of the Government Chemist where they were bulked, freeze dried and examined for protein, fat, ash, calcium, iron, sodium, potassium, thiamin, riboflavin, nicotinic acid, vitamin B_6, folic acid and essential fatty and amino acids. The results, most of which are summarised in Table 2, show that, in general, there are

TABLE 2

COMPARISON OF THE NUTRIENT CONTENT OF BREAD PRODUCED BY
THE CHORLEYWOOD BREAD PROCESS AND BY CONVENTIONAL MEANS

| Nutrients/100 g | Bread produced by | |
	Chorleywood process	Conventional method
Moisture (g)	39·0	38·5
Protein (N × 5·7) (g)	8·0	8·4
Fat (g)	1·7	1·7
Calcium (mg)	100	100
Iron (mg)	1·7	1·8
Sodium (mg)	540	540
Potassium (mg)	100	100
Thiamin (mg)	0·18	0·18
Riboflavin (mg)	0·03	0·02
Available nicotinic acid (mg)	0·82	0·83
Total nicotinic acid (mg)	1·43	1·40
Vitamin B_6 (μg)	40	40
Folic acid (*L. casei*) (μg)	6	6

Reference: Knight *et al.* (1973).

no great differences between the two types of retail white bread and that the values are similar to those found by Chamberlain *et al.* (1966) for those nutrients then determined, with the exception of thiamin which, in the more recent study, shows less difference between the two baking processes. Essential fatty and amino acids also showed little difference between the two types of loaves. The content of riboflavin was slightly higher and of protein slightly lower in the CBP bread than in conventional

TABLE 3

MEAN RESULTS FOR COMPOSITION OF TWO MUSCLES OF BEEF CATTLE EXTENSIVELY AND INTENSIVELY REARED

Muscle	Treatment	Moisture (%)	Fat (%)	Protein (%)	Iron (mg/100 g)	Thiamin (mg/100 g)	Riboflavin (mg/100 g)	Nicotinic acid (mg/100 g)
Longissimus dorsi	Extensive	71·8	5·2	22·1	1·82	0·05	0·13	7·36
	Intensive	72·3	3·8	22·1	1·64	0·07	0·15	6·79
Superficial digital flexor	Extensive	72·2	4·5	21·8	2·89	0·05	0·16	4·04
	Intensive	73·6	3·1	21·2	2·68	0·08	0·18	5·16

Reference: Harries *et al.* (1968).

bread but none of the differences were of nutritional significance. Full details of the study will soon appear in the British Journal of Nutrition (Knight *et al.*, 1973).

BEEF AND MEAT PRODUCTS

The practice of rearing beef cattle on diets with a high barley content has raised the question of the nutritive values of such intensively produced beef. To obtain information about this Harries *et al.* (1968) examined samples of lean raw beef from animals that had been intensively and extensively reared at three research institutes. Determinations were made of the moisture, fat, protein, iron, thiamin, riboflavin and nicotinic acid contents of two muscles—*longissimus dorsi* and superficial *digital flexor*. Some representative results taken from their paper are given in Table 3 from which it is apparent that there are no significant differences between intensively reared and extensively reared animals in respect of this range of nutrients. An examination was also made of pieces of liver from the region adjacent to the gall bladder for vitamins B_6, B_{12}, folic acid, vitamin A and carotene in addition to those nutrients determined on the samples of beef. Some results are given in Table 4 from which the authors concluded that there was less vitamin A and less carotene in samples of liver from intensively reared animals than in comparable samples from extensively reared animals.

The processing of canned meats had undergone considerable technological advances, the pumping of brine into hams has resulted in a moister product with a corresponding decrease in the protein content. The more recent process of tumbling meat eliminates the need for binders to bind the meat segments but increases the moisture retention properties of the meat. Ascorbic acid is added as an antioxidant; after processing the canned meat products contain nutritionally significant amounts of ascorbic acid. Recent samples of European origin have an ascorbic acid content of 40 mg/100 g. EEC legislation appears to be based on the concept that the meat used in the production of canned meat should be restricted to skeletal meat. The UK law permits the use of offal and if the EEC approach is adopted it would appear likely that the B vitamin content of canned meats will be reduced.

EGGS

The management of the laying hen has undergone great changes in the last decade so that by 1971 the proportion of birds maintained in battery conditions had risen to almost 85% whereas for other intensive systems

TABLE 4

MEAN RESULTS FOR NUTRIENTS IN LIVER OF BEEF CATTLE EXTENSIVELY AND INTENSIVELY REARED

Treatment	Moisture (%)	Fat (%)	Protein (%)	Iron (mg/100 g)	Thiamin (mg/100 g)	Riboflavin (mg/100 g)	Nicotinic acid (mg/100 g)	Vit. B_6 (mg/100 g)	Vit. B_{12} (μg/100 g)	Folic acid (μg/100 g)	Vit. A (iu/100 g)	Carotene (ppm)
Extensive	71·0	1·3	19·5	3·6	0·17	2·68	13·0	0·76	105	148	37 000	9·8
Intensive	69·4	3·7	21·2	5·0	0·15	2·71	13·1	0·81	93	148	13 000	<0·5
Intensive	70·8	3·1	21·2	5·8	0·19	2·64	13·1	1·11	58	143	100	<0·5

Reference: Harries *et al.* (1968).

including deep litter the proportion had fallen to 10 % and for the free
range system to less than 6 %. Such changes have been accompanied by
much discussion about the possibility of a deterioration in the nutritional
quality of eggs, which has tended to become obscured by views on the
general acceptability of eggs in terms of their palatability, yolk colour and
physical characteristics. Little information on the comparative composition
of eggs obtained under different systems of management has been published.
Therefore a study was initiated by the Committee on Food Composition
to obtain data on the composition of eggs representative of those available
to the consumer. Monthly samples of 18 eggs from birds maintained under
battery, deep litter and free range conditions were supplied for 15 months
by 6 agricultural institutes and colleges throughout the United Kingdom.

TABLE 5

MEAN VALUE FOR NUTRIENT CONTENT OF EGGS PER 100 g EDIBLE WEIGHT

Nutrient	Battery	Deep litter	Free range
Moisture (g)	74·7	75·1	74·6
Fat (g)	10·9	10·7	11·1
Protein (N × 6·25) (g)	12·3	12·2	12·4
Calcium (mg)	55	51	51
Iron (mg)	2·06	1·93	2·08
Sodium (mg)	139	139	136
Potassium (mg)	135	134	138
Thiamin (mg)	0·091	0·088	0·090
Riboflavin (mg)	0·47	0·50	0·45
Nicotinic acid (mg)	0·068	0·065	0·070
Pantothenic acid (mg)	1·7	1·8	1·8
Folic acid:			
(*Strep. faecalis*) (μg)	6	10	9
(*L. casei*) (μg)	25	32	39
Vitamin B_{12} (μg)	1·7	2·6	2·9
Tocopherols (mg)	1·5	1·8	1·5
Retinol (μg)	140	138	145

Reference: Tolan *et al.* (1973).

After storage at 10° to 13°C for 14 days after lay (the average age of an
egg when purchased by the consumer) the eggs were homogenised, freeze
dried in the laboratory and kept at −15° until required for analysis. The
freeze-dried material was examined for the following constituents: nitrogen,
fat, calcium, iron, sodium, potassium, cholesterol, vitamin A (retinol),
carotenoid pigments, thiamin, riboflavin, nicotinic acid, pantothenic acid,
folic acid, vitamin B_{12}, tocopherols, amino and fatty acids. Some of the
results obtained, taken from Tolan *et al.* (1973), are given in Table 5.

For most of the nutrients little difference was found between the composition of the eggs from the three systems of management. Statistically significant differences occurred in some vitamins, notably folic acid and vitamin B_{12}, both of which were lower in battery eggs than in eggs from the other management systems. Nutritionally these differences are of little significance in a mixed diet but for some individuals who may largely depend on eggs as a source of these vitamins such differences would be measurable. The amino and fatty acid composition of the eggs agreed with other published values and were unaffected by the system of management.

POTATOES

In Britain potatoes provide 28 % of the dietary intake of ascorbic acid and 13 % of the thiamin intake; they are therefore an important source of vitamin C and a useful one of thiamin. Consequently any loss of either vitamin as a result of processing could be of nutritional significance. The proportion of potatoes which are processed for human consumption increased in this country from about 2·5 % in 1955 to 11 % in 1969 and this trend is expected to continue for some years. The Committee on Food Composition decided therefore to conduct a small study on the vitamin content of some potato products and arranged for samples of potato powder, prepeeled potatoes and canned potatoes to be examined at the Laboratory of the Government Chemist for their content of vitamin C (ascorbic and dehydroascorbic acid), thiamin, sulphite and, for canned potatoes, folic

TABLE 6

VITAMIN CONTENT OF POTATO POWDER BEFORE RECONSTITUTION

Sample	Moisture (%)	Sulphur dioxide (ppm)	Vitamin C (mg/100 g)		Thiamin (mg/100 g)
			Total[a]	Reduced[b]	
Unfortified powder A	6·3	240	3·0	—	0·06
Unfortified powder B	9·7	550	14·0	10·0	<0·01
Unfortified powder C	5·7	140	9·8	9·5	0·06
Unfortified powder D	5·3	430	15·8	14·2	0·03
Unfortified flakes	5·9	550	4·2	3·5	0·02
Fortified powder A	—	—	—	158	—
Fortified powder B	—	—	—	161	—
Fortified powder C	—	—	—	117	—
Fortified powder D	—	—	—	185	—

[a] Ascorbic, dehydroascorbic and dioxogulonic acids.

[b] Ascorbic acid.

acid. Some typical results showing the levels of the vitamins present in
potato powder and prepeeled potatoes are given in Tables 6 and 7; results
of storage trials on the vitamin content of canned potatoes are given
in Table 8. When newly harvested, potatoes contain about 30 mg of
ascorbic acid/100 g, a value which falls to 8 mg/100 g after storage for
9 months. It is apparent from results in Table 6 that considerable destruction of ascorbic acid occurs during the production of potato powder and

TABLE 7

VITAMIN CONTENT OF COMMERCIALLY PEELED AND CHIPPED POTATOES

	Moisture (%)	Sulphur dioxide (ppm)	Vitamin C (mg/100 g)		Thiamin (mg/100 g)
			Total[a]	Reduced[b]	
Chipped potatoes	82	320	7·5	7·4	0·06
Peeled potatoes (small)	78	415	7·3	7·5	0·04
Peeled potatoes (large)	—	—	7·6	7·0	—

[a] Ascorbic, dehydroascorbic and dioxogulonic acids.
[b] Ascorbic acid.

that the thiamin content is greatly reduced probably owing to the use of
sulphite as a preserving agent. To compensate for the loss of ascorbic acid
some manufacturers now add ascorbic acid to their product in amounts
approximately equivalent to that present in new potatoes as shown by the
values for fortified powders given in Table 6. Prepeeled potatoes and chips
were found to contain at most 10 mg of vitamin C/100 g, a value similar
to that found in potatoes stored for 7 months (Table 7). On the other hand
losses of vitamin C from potatoes that had been harvested, processed and
canned on the same day were small and little change occurred on storage
of the canned product for 30 months (Table 8).

SOME CURRENT DEVELOPMENTS

Many supermarkets now carry up to ten times the number of food items
displayed a decade ago. The food industry, to meet consumer demands
and to produce competitive products, has introduced a number of products
which involve the replacement of conventional foods or their ingredients,
by products which may not be nutritionally equivalent.

Convenience foods
The descriptive but ill-defined title of 'convenience foods' is applied to
meals or meal components which require a minimum of preparation or

TABLE 8

VITAMIN CONTENT OF CANNED POTATOES AFTER STORAGE AT 5°C FOR 6 MONTHS AND THEREAFTER AT 20°C

Canning process	9·5 minutes at 260°F					30 minutes at 240°F				
Storage time (months)	0	3	6	12	30	0	3	6	12	30
Thiamin (mg/100 g)										
solids	0·041	0·037	0·049	0·033	0·028	0·037	0·031	0·038	0·033	0·031
liquids	0·030	0·045	0·044	0·037	0·035	0·029	0·039	0·043	0·037	0·033
Vitamin C (mg/100 g)										
[a]total—solids	21	24	22	20	23	18	19	21	20	21
[a]total—liquid	20	25	24	23	22	19	21	24	23	23
[b]reduced—solids	17	23	21	20	21	19	19	22	20	19
[b]reduced—liquid	—	26	21	23	23	18	21	23	23	23
Folic acid (μg/100 g)										
[c]total—solids	—	70	73	60	50	—	66	70	55	50
[c]total—liquid	—	67	79	48	40	—	53	57	43	55
[d]free—solids	—	1	1	1	1	—	1	2	1	1
[d]free—liquid	—	1	1	1	1	—	1	1	1	1

[a] Ascorbic, dehydroascorbic and dioxogulonic acids.
[b] Ascorbic acid.
[c] L. casei assay for conjugate and non-conjugate folates.
[d] L. casei assay for non-conjugate folates.

cooking before consumption. Such products are of considerable interest to not only institutional and other large scale feeding establishments but already enjoy an increasing domestic market. One type of product which has been introduced recently is the high density main course meal, products which consist essentially of rice or some other form of carbohydrate, fish or meat with a sauce or condiment such as curry. A recent study (Armed Forces Food Services, 1972) compared commercial products available on the Australian market with typical conventional meals. Whilst they were equivalent in energy content the protein, ascorbic acid and thiamin contents of the convenience meals were significantly lower than the conventional meals. The average protein content was only 55 %, the ascorbic acid 12 % and the thiamin 60 % of the corresponding nutrients in the conventional meal, the major part of the energy content of the meal being derived from cereal adjuncts.

Unsaturated fatty acids

Whether or not the consumer should be advised to eat a higher proportion of unsaturated fats many conventional products are now available in which the animal fat is fully or partially replaced by unsaturated fats. Margarine is now available in which all fats are blended with oils rich in unsaturated fats. The total fatty acids of such products may contain up to 50 % of fatty acids of the unsaturated type and one third linoleic acid. Similarly there has been a displacement of animal fats used for frying by vegetable oils such as maize oil. In this context it is interesting to note that lard produced from pigs which have been fed on a diet consisting predominately of maize contains significant amounts of unsaturated fatty acid but its oily consistency makes it unsuitable for putting up in paper packs. To overcome this difficulty the lard is partially hydrogenated or hydrogenated lard flakes are added.

Dietary fibre

The foods consumed in the United Kingdom are not particularly rich in plant foods or high extraction cereal flours. In many composite products even the low extraction flours are being replaced by cereal starch devoid of fibre so that the total fibre intake is being further decreased. There is now evidence that an increased intake of dietary fibre is of clinical value in the treatment of disease of the colon. The present state of knowledge is insufficient to establish which component or whether all components of the plant cell wall are of clinical value.

Fructose

Food grade fructose is now commercially available and since this sugar at low temperature is approximately twice as sweet as sucrose it is now possible to halve the sugar content of many food products. The higher

TABLE 9

NOVEL PROTEINS

(Results on samples as received)

	Field bean			Soya									Raw lean beef
	1	2	3	1	2	3	4	5	6	7	8	9	
Moisture (%)	43·8	52·9	56·0	6·92	5·30	7·95	9·78	4·11	5·73	7·44	5·55	7·30	74·0
Nitrogen (%)	4·44	3·65	3·32	8·10	10·9	8·36	8·20	8·81	10·4	8·43	8·85	8·10	3·25
Protein (N × 6·25) (g)	27·7	22·8	20·8	50·6	68·0	52·3	51·3	55·1	65·0	52·7	55·3	50·6	20·2
Fat (%)	28·0	22·0	19·8	0·48	0·11	1·3	0·65	0·70	0·14	0·12	0·56	0·75	4·63
Ash (%)	0·15	0·65	1·4	5·9	4·3	5·9	6·0	6·2	10·1	6·3	6·3	10·9	—
Carbohydrate (by difference)	0·35	1·65	2·0	36·1	22·3	32·6	32·3	33·9	19·0	33·4	32·3	30·4	
Calcium (mg/100 g)	11·2	12·9	15·4	230	230	230	240	240	200	320	260	260	13·0
Iron (mg/100 g)	6·0	5·1	5·7	16	11	9·2	9·4	19	11	10	9·8	8·0	2·1
Sodium (mg/100 g)	6	240	500	23	1 090	5	5	20	2 250	30	4	8·0	62
Potassium (mg/100 g)	2	6	5	2 280	560	2 280	2 260	2 350	1 340	2 370	2 460	2 150	345
Magnesium (mg/100 g)	0·9	1·9	2·2	290	110	290	290	300	200	290	300	260	20
Zinc (mg/100 g)	2·5	1·4	1·5	5·2	5·1	5·5	5·4	5·8	3·3	5·4	5·8	5·4	4·3
Copper (mg/100 g)	0·69	0·72	0·54	1·8	2·2	1·9	1·7	1·9	1·3	1·7	2·2	1·8	0·14
Chloride (mg/100 g)	38	360	740	13	320	12	16	14	3 400	36	14	3 180	59
Phosphorus (mg/100 g)	20	170	150	640	640	640	590	660	570	630	680	630	179
Thiamin (mg/100 g)	0·01	2·5	0·01	1·4	0·15	0·98	0·74	2·0	0·34	0·72	0·70	0·77	0·07
Riboflavin (mg/100 g)	0·03	0·10	0·01	2·3	0·34	0·36	0·36	2·1	0·55	0·35	1·4	0·32	0·24
Nicotinic acid (mg/100 g)	<0·1	0·12	<0·1	29	0·90	2·4	2·3	30	6·3	2·2	18	2·9	5·2
Vitamin B$_6$ (mg/100 g)	0·01	0·01	0·01	2·6	0·23	0·81	0·75	3·7	0·94	0·77	1·8	0·73	0·32
Vitamin B$_{12}$ (µg/100 g)	1	<1	<1	10	<1	<1	<1	12	4	<1	13	<1	2
Folic acid non-conjugate L. casei (µg/100 g)	3	2	<1	20	34	27	22	32	18	27	31	33	4
Pantothenic acid (mg/100 g)	0·17	0·15	0·07	3·9	1·3	2·3	2·2	6·5	1·6	1·9	3·4	2·1	0·68
Biotin (µg/100 g)	5	4	4	33	38	39	37	42	22	32	41	33	<1

TABLE 10

NOVEL PROTEINS

(mg amino acid/g nitrogen)

	Field bean			Soya									Raw lean beef
	1	2	3	1	2	3	4	5	6	7	8	9	
Alanine	250	250	260	260	260	250	260	260	270	230	250	260	390
Arginine	550	550	530	400	400	420	430	470	480	390	420	410	420
Aspartic acid	740	740	730	710	710	720	720	700	710	670	710	700	580
Cystine	50	50	50	90	90	110	120	90	90	100	100	100	80
Glutamic acid	1 150	1 180	1 230	1 230	1 240	1 230	1 240	1 250	1 310	1 170	1 250	1 270	1 040
Glycine	250	250	250	250	250	250	250	250	250	220	250	240	350
Histidine	190	190	220	210	210	200	200	200	200	200	200	190	230
Isoleucine	310	310	300	280	280	290	290	270	270	280	270	280	310
Leucine	520	520	520	450	450	440	440	440	440	420	460	450	480
Lysine	500	510	500	470	470	470	470	470	470	470	440	440	550
Methionine	50	50	50	90	90	90	90	90	80	90	90	90	160
Phenylalanine	320	320	330	290	280	320	320	300	320	300	310	300	280
Proline	300	300	310	330	330	340	350	300	300	320	330	330	320
Serine	370	370	380	360	360	370	370	360	370	340	350	360	280
Threonine	240	240	240	250	250	260	260	240	240	230	260	260	270
Tryptophan	60	60	60	80	80	70	80	80	80	80	80	80	80
Tyrosine	230	230	230	180	190	200	200	210	200	190	200	190	240
Valine	340	350	340	330	330	300	310	330	320	270	320	300	320

relative sweetness of fructose is likely to lead to the replacement of sorbitol in diabetic foods. However, Macdonald (1970) has suggested that the fructose moiety of the sucrose molecule is responsible for increasing the triglyceride level of blood serum. If this view is correct then the displacement of sucrose and other sugar by fructose is not without significance.

Novel proteins
No consideration of future trends would be complete without considering the impact of the use of novel proteins on food composition. Recently, the Laboratory of the Government Chemist, on behalf of the Committee on Medical Aspects of Food Policy, examined a range of texturised vegetable proteins. The results, most of which are summarised in Tables 9 and 10, show that when compared with raw meat there are significant differences in the levels of B vitamins, levels of inorganic nutrients and the distribution of amino acids, particularly methionine. Several samples of each type were tested for vitamin A and carotene but neither was detected. Ascorbic acid did not exceed 1 mg/100 g; no appreciable amounts of tocopherols were found in the soya products. Samples of the products based on field bean protein contained 3 μg/g of α-tocopherol and 8 μg/g γ-tocopherol.

FOOD ADDITIVES

In this paper no detailed consideration has been given to the effect on food composition of chemicals which are intentionally or inadvertently added to human foods during processing. It is difficult to assess the overall situation. These are matters which internationally are the concern of the World Health Organization and the Codex Alimentarius Committee on Food Additives, and a start has been made by WHO to estimate the food additive intake. Further studies have been recommended by the Joint FAO/WHO Expert Committee on Food Additives to assess high persistent consumption of additives by individuals.

CONCLUSION

In conclusion, surveys with the aim of assessing the effects of modern methods of animal husbandry and food processing on the nutrient content of food are subject to several limitations. New techniques usually involve a number of changes in the conventional process which make it difficult to isolate the effect of a single variable. Direct comparison of the product from new and traditional processes are also not easy to arrange for both methods are seldom in operation under normal commercial conditions at one site. In addition, if samples are collected at the retail outlet there is uncertainty about their identity unless special arrangements can be made. Even so, within these limitations, it has been possible to obtain useful information on the effects of processing on the composition of some important items of food.

Studies of chicken, bread, beef, eggs and potatoes have shown no pronounced losses of major nutrients except in two instances—the substantial destruction of vitamin C during the production of potato powder and the low value of retinol found in the liver of intensively reared cattle. The loss of vitamin C in potato powder is the more serious and it is reassuring to find that some manufacturers are now adding vitamin C to their product to restore that loss in processing. Other vitamins such as thiamin, folic acid and vitamin B_{12} have shown some fluctuations in chicken meat, eggs and potatoes but none was of nutritional significance when considered as part of a mixed diet.

Equally the other changes in food composition described as future trends are unlikely to be of nutritional significance in a mixed diet but more detailed information is needed. This should, in some instances, be based on the examination of a larger number of samples for a wider range of nutrients. There is a continuing need to keep the composition of new foods under review.

REFERENCES

Armed Forces Food Services (1972). *Value of High Density Convenience Foods*, report no. 3. Establishment Commonwealth of Australia.
Chamberlain, N., Collins, T. H., Elton, G. A. H., Hollingsworth, D. F., Lisle, D. B. and Payne, P. R. (1966). *Br. J. Nutr.*, **20,** 747.
Harries, J. M., Hubbard, A. W., Alder, F. E., Kay, M. and Williams, D. R. (1968). *Br. J. Nutr.*, **22,** 21.
Knight, R. A., Christie, A. A., Orton, C. R. and Robertson, J. (1973). *Br. J. Nutr.* In press.
Macdonald, I. (1970). In *Glucose Syrups and Related Carbohydrates*, p. 86, edited by G. G. Birch, L. F. Green and C. B. Coulson, Applied Science, London.
Robertson, J., Vipond, M. S., Tapsfield, D. and Greaves, J. P. (1966). *Br. J. Nutr.*, **20,** 675.
Tolan, A., Robertson, J., Orton, C. R., Christie, A. A. and Millburn, B. A. (1973). *Br. J. Nutr.* In press.

CHAPTER 25

Health and 'health foods'

H. M. SINCLAIR

Magdalen College, Oxford

THE THREE AGES OF MAN'S FOODS

This symposium is concerned with nutritional problems in changing Britain, today and tomorrow. To assess the relation of the food industry to 'health foods', I must briefly look at yesterday.

When we crept in primordial slime, we engulfed protein that we happened to contact. Later we moved towards attractive chemicals, just as today the unicellular slime-mould (*Dictyostelium discoideum*) is attracted by cyclic-AMP produced by live *E. coli*. If this food is not available, the mould itself secretes the chemical, attracting other slime moulds to it and so forming a multicellular organism. Today we still use cyclic-AMP, but as an internal secondary messenger, and an omniscient slime-mould might regard us as becoming a multicellular organism on Saturday afternoons. Eyes and noses enabled us to select foods, and for the major part of his existence man has been a food gatherer, first eating fruits, nuts and berries with occasional small animals, later with the aid of tools hunting and eating large animals including his own species.

The second period was reached some 8000 years ago when with the introduction of agriculture man became a food producer. But failure of crops, as through drought and poor methods of storage or preparation, caused frequent famines.

In the last half century man has been entering upon his third and most significant period, that of food manufacturer. The rise of modern food technology, which I do not intend to discuss, has obviously depended largely upon advances in the sciences of chemistry and nutrition, but drawn also from others such as microbiology and physics. Before mentioning its relation to health and 'health foods', I must define the words we are using.

WHAT ARE 'HEALTH FOODS'?

I have recently discussed in some detail elsewhere (Sinclair, 1972) the definition and the origin of the concept of a 'health food', and the inadequate definitions given by some recent writers. The two words embrace for most people, I suspect, two different concepts. The first is that the food contains all the nutrients originally present in the natural foodstuff, except those inevitably lost in necessary processes of preparation. The second is that no harmful substance has been added to the food in the course of preparing it from the natural foodstuff or in the course of producing that foodstuff. It is irrelevant where the food is sold or even if it is sold. An orange is a health food although not normally sold in a health food shop; if a colouring agent added to the peel gets into the fruit and is toxic, the orange ceases to be a health food. A lettuce grown in one's back garden is a health food unless it contains harmful amounts of additives such as pesticides.

But let us look a little more closely at the orange. Strictly, it is not a food at all unless the peel is used as for marmalade: otherwise, it is a foodstuff. This is a substance that may be treated to form food, and a food is what is ingested by the organism and provides one or more aliments and nutrients (Sinclair, 1948). Suppose we take a litre of water, add 1 g of ascorbic acid, a permitted synthetic orange dye and some decanol, we might have an imitation orange juice that might deceive the consumer and in one respect be a superior food to natural orange juice in that the content of ascorbic acid would be about twice that found naturally. In terms of Atwaters (Sinclair, 1949; these nutritional units are explained below), 100 g of orange juice contains: ascorbic acid, 68; thiamin, 2·8; calcium, 1·8; iron, 1·6; carbohydrate, 1·4; all other major nutrients are below 1·0. But there are minor nutrients and other substances that might be nutritionally important: orange juice contains seven other vitamins of the B complex, seventeen carotenoids, eleven flavonoids, eleven amino acids, also pectins and protopectins, enzymes and more than 50 aromatic flavouring components. Of course these may be irrelevant, but orange juice is a rich source of 'vitamin P' (Rusznýak and Szent-Györgyi, 1936) which allegedly includes flavonones such as eriodictyol and hesperitin. But in orthodox circles it is not a nutrient. However, some consider it has not definitely been excluded from this category, and if they are right our imitation orange juice could not be a health food. Certainly flavonoids require more study, in relation to their antioxidant properties (Clemetson and Andersen, 1966), their known effect on cancer cells and their metabolism (De Eds, 1968).

Sucrose is certainly a food: 100 g provides nearly 1650 kJ (for nutritionists of yesterday, 400 kcal; for those of tomorrow, 22 Atwaters). But it is not a health food: certain nutrients, such as pyridoxine and chromium, are removed during manufacture, and the presence of the former of these might account for the absence of dental caries in Jamaicans and Cubans who suck sugar cane.

White flour, about 70% extraction and bleached with chlorine dioxide, is a food but certainly not a health food, despite the two vitamins and two salts that are added. I have discussed elsewhere (Sinclair, 1958) the possible importance of some nutrients that are mainly removed (such as essential fatty acids and pyridoxine) or destroyed (such as tocopherols). At this Conference Mr Burkitt has discussed the importance of fibre (Burkitt, 1972). In 1955 Sir Henry (now Lord) Cohen and his Panel were asked to determine nutritional differences between national flour and flour of lower extraction with or without three token nutrients. They decided (Cohen, 1956) that it was 'important that the flour should be as nutritious as possible'; but they differed from the Government's medical and scientific advisers and the Medical Research Council in that they concluded that there was no ascertainable difference between flour of lower extraction to which thiamin, nicotinic acid and iron had been restored, and national flour, 'which would significantly affect the health of the population in any foreseeable circumstances'. They thought it very unlikely that lowering the extraction rate from 80% to 70% would lead to any nutritional disturbance from lack of pyridoxine. The two commonest (indeed, almost universal) nutritional disturbances in this country are atherosclerosis and dental caries. Monkeys deficient in pyridoxine develop these two disorders (Rinehart and Greenberg, 1956); Dr Rinehart and his colleagues did large numbers of estimations of human plasma transaminase, rarely found them maximal and in these cases regularly obtained a 30 to 100% increase by administration of pyridoxine. Very low plasma values for coenzyme forms of pyridoxine have been found in patients with coronary atherosclerosis (Gvozdova et al., 1966). A controlled trial on 540 US pregnant women showed that adminstration of pyridoxine decreased dental caries and increased serum transaminase (Hillman et al., 1962). Various studies have shown that women taking the contraceptive pill may require as much as 30 mg of pyridoxine daily (Luhby et al., 1971; Brin, 1971). Using the figures of Cohen (1956) and of Hollingsworth et al. (1956), it seemed that the per caput daily consumption of pyridoxine in Britain was about 1·7 mg on national flour (which provided about 40% of the dietary pyridoxine) and 1·3 mg on 70% extraction flour, and I concluded (Sinclair, 1958) that some of us 'have viewed with some alarm the relatively low per caput consumption of this important vitamin even when flour of 80% extraction was in general use'. Coppock (quoted by Sinclair, 1972) has stated in relation to flour: 'The nutrients that the health food people say are taken out are in fact restored'. This is not true of pyridoxine since 72% extraction flour has lost 70% of that in wholemeal, and this nutrient urgently needs increased attention in our diets. Nor is Coppock's statement true of any other vitamin of the B complex, except thiamin and nicotinic acid which are added by law to all flour (Parliament, 1956).

It should be mentioned that we do not understand adequately why deficiency of a nutrient can cause very different clinical syndromes. Deficiency of pyridoxine can cause dermatosis or peripheral neuropathy or normocytic anaemia. The biochemical causes of the lesions produced by nutrient deficiencies, either alone or in combination, require much more investigation. The recent studies of Schroeder (1971) emphasise that deficiencies may occur more easily than we suppose through processing and sophistication of foods: 'These data demonstrate the dietary needs for the use of whole grains and unprocessed foods of most varieties. They suggest that enrichment of refined flours, sugars, and fats with some vitamins and essential trace elements may be necessary to meet recommended daily allowances, especially of vitamin B_6, pantothenic acid, chromium, zinc and possibly manganese'.

FOODS FOR HEALTH

We, like the slime-mould, must have foods to keep us healthy. Aliments and nutrients must be neither deficient nor excessive. We now have very detailed knowledge about these limits, but there is still much to learn, particularly about the long-term effects of either. Excesses are perhaps more important than is customarily supposed. Ascorbic acid is partly oxidised to oxalate, and it may not have been just a coincidence that a patient of whom I have knowledge was given large amounts of ascorbic acid daily after a severe myocardial infarct to avoid infections, but died during surgery for oxalate stones which he had not previously experienced. Twenty years ago Dr Lloyd and I called attention to the work of Scheunert (1949) on the positive effect of supplements on the health of factory workers, and concluded that 'It would be well worth while to conduct further large-scale experiments of this type' (Lloyd and Sinclair, 1953). Since then conflicting trials have been carried out, but two recent ones have claimed favourable results of massive amounts (Charleston and Clegg, 1972; Anderson et al., 1972). But we must remember that ascorbic acid increases absorption of iron, and haemosiderosis can be fatal.

Absolute amounts in the food are not all that concerns us. Schroeder (1968), for instance, has called attention to the variations in availability of dietary sources of chromium, and differences in this respect between refined and crude sugar. The unknown cause of the relation of hardness of drinking water to cardiovascular disease (Crawford, 1972) illustrates our remarkable ignorance of important dietary factors, and the need for caution in our practices as for instance softening water supplies.

But there is more to food than content, balance and availability of aliments and nutrients. Taste, smell, freshness and attractiveness are factors of which we understand little. Meals are becoming less important as social occasions. Man is a herd animal, like the dog and unlike the cat. Instinctively he eats with other members of the herd. He has become accustomed to using meals for ritual purposes—the wedding breakfast, the christening cake, funeral meats, regimental or club dinners, the tribal feast, social teas, the family midday Sunday meal with the householder carving the joint. These will continue but the pattern of ordinary eating is altering and will alter further with informal snacks replacing formal meals.

The provision of snacks will alter. There has been an evolution from the village store, through the grocery shop to the supermarket, which will soon be replaced by cash-and-carry centres until these are superseded by direct delivery into the deep-freeze. From this will be taken a complete snack that only needs thawing and perhaps warming in the living room, for the kitchen is becoming obsolete. Prepacked meals therefore need a long shelf-life, and this causes alterations in composition either from destruction of nutrients or addition of chemical substances. Essential fatty acids, easily destroyed with production of rancid flavours unless a powerful antioxidant is present, are perhaps more vulnerable than other nutrients.

LABELLING OF FOODS

Purchasers have a right to know what is contained in the foods they purchase, both the nutrients that remain and the chemical compounds that are added. There then remains the problem of indirect food additives, for instance contamination from food film wraps. DEHP (di-2-ethylhexyl phthalate) is one such, but is becoming restricted to foods of high water content, and a commoner substance is now DOA (di-(2-ethylhexyl)adipate). Lake Superior now contains 300 ppb DEHP, and certain fish in the Mississipi River more than ten times this (*Food Chemical News*, 1973). Perhaps this is unimportant, but more studies of teratogenicity are needed.

The Food and Drugs Act, 1955, specifies that under usual circumstances it is an offence to sell 'to the prejudice of the purchaser any food or drug which is not of the nature, or not of the substance, or not of the quality, of the food or drug demanded by the purchaser'. About eight Statutory Instruments dealing with labelling have subsequently been produced, of which the two most recent are the Labelling of Food Regulations 1970 (SI 1970/400) and the Labelling of Food (Amendment) Regulations 1972 (SI 1972/1510).

Very recently in the USA the Food and Drug Administration of the Department of Health, Education, and Welfare has introduced very detailed proposals for 'food labeling' that occupy over 40 pages of the *Federal Register* for 19 January 1973 (Food and Drug Administration, 1973). An interesting new departure is the labelling of foods in relation to cholesterol and to fat and fatty acids, 'polyunsaturated fatty acids' being specified as meaning those that are *cis*, *cis*-methylene-interrupted (and therefore presumably essential fatty acids), and 'saturated fatty acids' as being the sum of C_{12} to C_{18}. The FDA proposed 'a standardized format for listing seven commonly analyzed nutrients' (five vitamins, iron and calcium; later it admitted it had overlooked protein), and proposed they be listed as a % of the US Recommended Dietary Allowances provided the figure is not less than 2% (equivalent to 2·86 Atwaters). At last the need for a nutritional unit has become appreciated in official circles.

This need has been obvious for decades. When early in the 1939–45 War the Oxford Nutrition Survey did repeated dietary analyses, we found errors could occur because there was no mental check that the figures were the right order of magnitude: if one states that a man is tall, namely 6000 feet high, one immediately notices an error; but if one tells a dietist that 100 g of dried apricots contain 5 mg of folic acid, she will not shudder at the similar thousand-fold error. She will only realise that the figure is preposterous if she reasons that the daily adult folate requirement is about 0·05 mg, therefore 1 g of dried apricots would provide the daily requirement, and she was not taught that this food was so admirable a source of this nutrient. We therefore drew up our food tables and calculated our diets in terms of a logical nutritional unit, the Atwater (Sinclair, 1949). We drew up weekly allowances for a moderately active woman for energy, aliments and nutrients, and the weights of these (or amounts of energy) were 1000 At for each factor. Thus, if we allow her 1 mg daily of a nutrient, 1 At of that nutrient is equal to $(1 \times 7)/1000$ mg. Less than 1 At is insignificant, so no decimals occur. It is obvious that she should obtain an average of 143 At of each factor daily (1000/7), so she can easily assess from a properly labelled food the value of that food in providing her energy and nutrients.

This objective food labelling would assist in ensuring that the public is informed and not misled. Long confusing names, incomprehensible units, false descriptions, misleading statements, should disappear. The statement that Blank's Breakfast Food 'contains appreciable quantities of unknown nutrients' may be true, but is misleading. The statement that each of Bilge's Beefburgers 'contains not less than 70 mg of cholesterol and cholesterol is good for you' may be true and the body needs cholesterol, but the statement is misleading. Fortunately we have the Advertising Standards Authority that supervises the Code of Advertising Practice Committee. For instance, 'Scientific jargon and irrelevancies should not be used to make claims appear to have a scientific basis they do not possess'. I regret that both the Advertising Standards Authority and the CAP Committee believe 'there is insufficient support from medical opinion to justify advertisement copy claims that health benefits will or may result if products, such as corn oils and margarine, containing a high proportion of polyunsaturated fats are substituted for fats of animal origin, e.g. butter and lard'. Scandinavian countries and Holland seem to be in advance of us in this respect.

The Code very properly condemns misuse of scientific terms, statistics or quotations. The Ministry of Health (1963) stated that 'It would be necessary to drink at one time $2\frac{1}{2}$ bathfuls of water containing fluoride at a concentration of 1 ppm before any harmful effects due to fluoride would be experienced'. Since this obviously referred to acute toxicity (Sinclair, 1964) which is irrelevant in discussing possible dangers from long-term ingestion, the Ministry's statement was, in my opinion, either intentionally misleading or just ignorant.

Ignorant or misleading statements should be quashed by facts whenever possible. Silly statements appear in support of health foods; dogmatic outbursts occur in opposition.

FOODS OF TOMORROW

We now know most of, but not all, the nutrients required by man, and the approximate amounts in many instances. This interesting knowledge has been acquired mainly in the last few years. I have pointed out elsewhere (Sinclair, 1972) how it could and should be put into practice by making available the nutrients (vitamins, minerals, essential fatty acids, essential amino acids or the corresponding fatty acids) in a convenient food such as a biscuit so that a person need only consume one daily to get his or her known nutrients. Then he or she could satisfy hunger and appetite, and thereby obtain energy, by eating whatever was desired and available, with no worries about nutrient requirements. Obesity could be easily controlled by simply eating less; the possible harm of some 3000 additives is watched by the Government.

The foods of tomorrow will be largely synthetic. Within the next 25 years—certainly the next half century—the bullock should become extinct and the cow confined to zoos. We can make much better 'beef steaks' from plant sources, although there are many problems, such as the loss of essential fatty acids in the phospholipids of animal cell membranes, loss of vitamin B_{12}, and the presence in plant fats of lipopolysaccharides and fatty acids with propane rings and branched chains that are absorbed and may enter brain phospholipids. We will not have to put plants through a cow to obtain milk—an imperfect food for man as produced by a cow—or through a hen to produce eggs—an imperfect food for man as produced from a battery hen. The nutritionist of tomorrow will realise that proteins, and even 'essential' amino acids, are not essential for man.

But even if all known nutrients are provided by nutribisks, synthetic foods raise a host of nutritional problems, as I have just indicated. The desire amongst the public for 'health foods' arises to a large extent from the fact that the great advances in food technology have taken place without the necessary human nutritional research being undertaken. As I have pointed out recently (Sinclair, 1972), it is quite wrong to hide behind a smoke screen of statements that we are better fed and healthier than ever before, when chronic degenerative diseases that are primarily nutritional in origin are very prevalent in a country such as ours and are increasing in incidence. Such diseases probably include dental caries, atherosclerosis and ischaemic heart disease, pulmonary embolism, certain forms of cancer, obesity, diabetes mellitus, senile osteoporosis, duodenal ulcers, cholelithiasis, acute appendicitis, diverticulosis, ulcerative colitis and Crohn's disease, varicose veins and haemorrhoids. The list could be extended, for instance, to include multiple sclerosis as a possibility. The rise in some of these diseases is halted by the national event of war, which suggests that these can be reversed by change in national diet. The rarity of these diseases in certain other countries provides clues to aetiology.

'BUSY COMMON SENSE'

At a conference in this University 16 years ago I quoted (Sinclair, 1958) from one of its greatest scientists and perhaps the greatest biologist since Darwin. Sir Charles Sherrington, asked 'what right have we to conjoin mental experience with physiological?' replied: 'No scientific right; only the right of what Keats, with that superlative Shakespearian gift of his, dubbed "busy common sense". The right which practical life, naïve and shrewd, often exercises. . . . Science, nobly, declines as proof anything but complete proof; but common sense, pressed for time, accepts and acts on acceptance'.

We do not have the nutritional knowledge to feed ourselves properly, and we are not demonstrably better fed and healthier than before in relation to chronic degenerative diseases. We see that there are countries in some respects better fed than we are. Lord Woolton witnessed that during the war we could become better fed in terms of health than before or probably after, and took the lead in establishing a central institute for research on human nutrition. This has now been established as a charitable organisation, the International Institute of Human Nutrition, to collect and integrate existing knowledge and to carry out research to try to fill some of the lamentable gaps in our knowledge.

Until we have more knowledge, common sense dictates that we should be humble enough to acknowledge that we do not know how to feed ourselves properly, and therefore the demand for 'health foods' will continue and increase. The future lies in human nutritional research and food technology advancing side by side, and then our teeming masses will become healthier and better fed than ever before, largely on man-made foods.

REFERENCES

Anderson, T. W., Reid, D. B. W. and Beaton, G. H. (1972). *Can. med. Ass. J.*, **107**, 503.

Brin, M. (1971). *Am. J. clin. Nutr.*, **24**, 699.

Burkitt, D. (1972). *Med. Ann.*, **90**, 5.

Charleston, S. S. and Clegg, K. M. (1972). *Lancet*, **1**, 1401.

Clemetson, C. A. B. and Andersen, L. (1966). *Ann. N.Y. Acad. Sci.*, **136**, 339.

Cohen, Sir H. (Chairman). (1956). *Report of the Panel on Composition and Nutritive Value of Flour* (Cmd. 9757). HMSO, London.

Crawford, M. D. (1972). *Proc. Nutr. Soc.*, **31**, 347.

De Eds, F. (1968). 'Flavonoid metabolism' in *Comprehensive Biochemistry*, **20**, pp. 127–171, edited by M. Florkin and E. H. Stotz, Elsevier, Amsterdam.

Food and Drug Administration (1973). *Fed. Reg.*, **38**, 2125.

Food Chemical News (1973). **15**, 38.

Gvozdova, L. G., Paramanova, E. G., Goryachenkova, E. V. and Polyakova, L. A. (1966). *Veprosy Pitanyia*, **25**, (4), 40.

Hillman, R. W., Cabaud, P. G. and Shenone, R. A. (1962). *Am. J. clin. Nutr.*, **10**, 512.

Hollingsworth, D. F., Vaughan, M. C. and Warnock, G. M. (1956). *Proc. Nutr. Soc.*, **15**, xvii.

Lloyd, B. B. and Sinclair, H. M. (1953). In *Biochemistry and Physiology of Nutrition*, pp. 369–471, edited by G. H. Bourne and G. W. Kidder, Academic Press, New York.

Luhby, A. L., Brin, M., Gordon, M., Davis, P., Murphy, M. and Spiegel, H. (1971). *Am. J. clin. Nutr.*, **24**, 684.

Ministry of Health (1963). *Fluoridation*, Ministry of Health, Alexander Fleming House, London.

Parliament. (1956). The Flour (Composition) Regulations (1956). *Stat. Instrum.* no. 1183.

Rinehart, J. F. and Greenberg, L. D. (1956). *Am. J. clin. Nutr.*, **4**, 318.

Rusznyák, S. and Szent-Györgyi, A. (1936). *Nature, Lond.*, **138**, 27.

Scheunert, A. (1949). *Int. Z. Vitaminforsch.*, **20**, 374.

Schroeder, H. A. (1968). *Am. J. clin. Nutr.*, **21**, 230.

Schroeder, H. A. (1971). *Am. J. clin. Nutr.*, **24**, 562.

Sinclair, H. M. (1948). *Vitam. Horm.*, **6**, 101.

Sinclair, H. M. (1949). *Br. J. Nutr.*, **3**, x.

Sinclair, H. M. (1958). *Proc. Nutr. Soc.*, **17**, 28.

Sinclair, H. M. (1964). *Br. med. J.*, **1**, 554.

Sinclair, H. M. (1972). In *Health and Food*, pp. 11–27, edited by G. G. Birch, L. F. Green and L. G. Plaskett, Applied Science, London.

CHAPTER 26

An industrialist's point of view

R. J. L. ALLEN

Group Research Director, Beecham Group Ltd, Brentford

THE INDUSTRY

The food industry is by definition deeply involved in nutrition. Food science and technology have enabled new public needs for food and sustenance to be met in changing political, economic and social circumstances which have transformed out of all recognition the way of life that prevailed before the Industrial Revolution. Without a large British food industry the urban population of this country could not be fed today. An enormous quantity of good quality sound food is produced and distributed at what are still by international standards competitive prices. In 1971 the weight of food moving into consumption in the United Kingdom (Table 1) was about 27 Tg (calculated from Ministry of Agriculture, Fisheries and Food, 1972a). Consumer expenditure on food amounted to £8041 m (Central Statistical Office, 1972), of which £5474 m (68%) (Food Manufacturers' Federation, 1972) was for manufactured foods (Table 2). The

TABLE 1

WEIGHT (Tg) OF FOOD MOVING INTO CONSUMPTION IN THE
UNITED KINGDOM IN 1971

Dairy products (not butter), as milk solids	1·40
Meat (including canned meat, bacon, ham), as edible weight	3·35
Fish, as edible weight	0·462
Eggs and egg products	0·854
Oils and fats (visible), fat content	1·24
Sugar and syrups, sugar content gross	2·88
Fruit (fresh equivalent)	3·22
Pulses and nuts	0·293
Potatoes	5·60
Other vegetables (fresh equivalent)	3·43
Grain products	4·03
Tea	0·207
Total	26·966

TABLE 2

CONSUMER EXPENDITURE (£m) ON MANUFACTURED FOODS
IN THE UNITED KINGDOM IN 1971

Grain milling	115
Bread and flour confectionery	648
Biscuits	211
Bacon curing, meat and fish products	1 206
Milk and milk products	1 248
Sugar	146
Cocoa, chocolate, sugar confectionery	497
Fruit and vegetable products	670
Vegetable and animal oils and fats	39
Soft drinks	243
Food industries not elsewhere specified	451
Total	5 474

TABLE 3

AMOUNTS OF ENERGY AND NUTRIENTS IN FOOD CONSUMED IN
PRIVATE HOUSEHOLDS IN THE UNITED KINGDOM IN 1969

Energy (TJ)	12 400 000
Protein (Gg)	1 510
Fat (Gg)	2 440
Carbohydrate (Gg)	6 440
Calcium (Mg)	21 300
Iron (Mg)	270
Thiamin (Mg)	23·8
Riboflavin (Mg)	36·4
Nicotinic acid equivalent (Mg)	598
Vitamin C (Mg)	1 050
Retinol equivalent (Mg)	27·8
Vitamin D (Mg)	0·0589

total amounts of energy and nutrients in food consumed in private house-
holds in 1969 as calculated from population statistics (Office of Population
Censuses and Surveys, 1972) and National Food Survey data (Ministry of
Agriculture, Fisheries and Food, 1971) are shown in Table 3.

ATTITUDES TO NUTRITION

There is today undoubtedly a greater general awareness among leaders
of the industry than ever before of the importance of nutrition and its
relevance to their commercial operations. The establishment, with industry
backing, of the British Nutrition Foundation in 1967, and indeed the fact
that this conference is being held, are evidence of that.

The newer knowledge of nutrition that developed in the early decades of
this century was applied between the wars in the production of such
products as infant foods and vitamin concentrates. However, I believe that
the present recognition of the significance of nutrition for the industry
stems mainly from the period of the Second World War and its aftermath.
It was then that many firms were compelled by circumstances to think
nutritionally about their problems. The evolution of national food policy,
primarily for defence reasons, made this inevitable. Rationing brought
with it a host of changes that required serious consideration to be given to
the nutritional value of the national food supply. Steps were taken as far
as possible to protect the consumer from the nutritional consequences of
wartime shortages and drastic changes in dietary patterns. Such measures
as the modification of the composition of bread and flour, the compulsory
addition of vitamins A and D to margarine and the provision of welfare
foods for nutritionally vulnerable population groups stem from this
period. The wartime vegetable dehydration industry in which many food
processing firms were engaged was established with a specific nutritional
objective (which was achieved): the nutritional value of the products was
to be not less than that of the equivalent cooked fresh vegetable (Allen
et al., 1944). Many of those involved in these projects are now in positions
of influence in the industry and the interest in nutrition that was generated
at that time is still being felt today.

All indications are that nutritional value is seldom the main factor in
determining consumer choice of foods. The housewife in the supermarket is
more likely to be influenced by price and palatability than by dietetic
considerations. Nevertheless in practical terms the food industry of
today recognises the need to pay due regard to modern nutritional thought
in the formulation, processing, packaging and distribution of its products.
To put it no higher, it can only be in the food manufacturer's own interests
to supply his customers with food that is safe and nutritious. Pressures
from governments and public opinion world wide are working in the same

direction and at the same time research is opening up new opportunities for those who are ready and equipped to respond. The influence of nutritional thought on the food industry can be seen today in many different areas. In the following paragraphs I discuss some of the more significant of these.

APPLICATIONS

Food processing

Davidson *et al.* (1972), in discussing food technology and nutrition, concluded that 'dependence on processed foods need reduce the nutritive value of the diet in no way'. Nevertheless the effects of food processing, transport and storage are rightly matters of continuing concern for food scientists and technologists. The factors that determine the nutritional value of processed foods have been comprehensively reviewed by Harris and von Loesecke (1960) and more recently by Hollingsworth and Martin (1972). There is a growing recognition of the joint role that food science and technology and nutrition must play in the maintenance and improvement of nutritional food quality.

Food fortification

Food fortification, which has been defined by the Joint FAO/WHO Expert Committee on Nutrition as the process whereby nutrients are added to foods to maintain or improve the quality of the diet (FAO/WHO, 1971), is another important area for the application of nutrition to food manufacture. The principles that should govern food fortification and the significance of this practice for public health nutrition are discussed in detail by the Committee in the same report. The bases on which nutrients can appropriately be added to food include to compensate for processing losses, or to ensure the nutritional quality of a substitute food, or as a technologically convenient and effective way of correcting a nutritional deficiency in the target population.

In the UK the only foods required by law to be fortified are flour (with calcium, iron, thiamin and nicotinic acid) and margarine (with vitamins A and D) but voluntary fortification is not uncommon, *e.g.* the addition of vitamin C to soft drinks and dried potato; thiamin, nicotinic acid and riboflavin to breakfast cereals; vitamins A and D to milk products; iodine to salt.

Foods for therapeutic purposes

Nutritional principles apply directly in the production of foods for use in diet therapy (Table 4). Some of these, for example sugar-free foods for diabetics and low sodium foods for use in cardiovascular disease, date back many years. With the rapid increase of our understanding of the

TABLE 4

COMMERCIALLY AVAILABLE FOODS FOR USE IN DIET THERAPY

Type	Indications
Carbohydrate-free or reduced foods in variety	Diabetes
Concentrated preparations of demineralised glucose and glucose polymers	Chronic renal insufficiency
Protein-free flour, bread, cakes, biscuits	
Amino acid mixtures	Acute renal insufficiency
Gluten-free flour, bread, cakes, biscuits	Gluten senstivity (coeliac disease)
Medium chain (C_8, C_{10}) triglyceride formulations	Hepatic dysfunction, fat intolerance
Low sodium foods in variety	Idiopathic hypertension, heart failure
Low lactose food	Disorders of carbohydrate metabolism
Low lactose/low fat food	
Reduced fat, low lactose food	
Sucrose and glucose-free food, fructose as sole source of carbohydrate	
Low phenylalanine casein hydrolysate	Disorders of protein metabolism
Formulated histidine-free foods	
Formulated foods with low phenylalanine, low tyrosine content and many others	
Formulated low calcium milks	Disorders of mineral metabolism (hypercalcaemia)
Arachis oil emulsions	Conditions requiring high energy, low fluid, low electrolyte diets
	Disorders of amino acid metabolism
Soya-based milk substitutes	Milk intolerance
Rapidly assimilable, nutritionally complete, residue-free formulations	Bowel fistulae and obstructions
	Inflammatory conditions of the digestive tract
Whole protein (calcium caseinate) formulations	Hypoproteinaemia
Nutritionally complete formulations for addition to milk or water	Conditions in which solid foods cannot be taken

biochemical lesions underlying many disease states, it has become possible more recently to formulate a whole range of new products that can be applied in the dietary management of specific disorders. In addition, nutritionally complete proprietary formulations are widely used for the preparation of liquid diets. Further advances in this area through coopera- tion between medical scientists and dietitians and food scientists can be expected.

Food additives

Many problems arising from the use of food additives are today regarded as the proper concern of nutritionists. Nutritional toxicology is rapidly becoming an important branch of nutritional science. Food additives are indispensable to modern food technology and play as significant a role in maintaining the food supply of industrialised societies as do the allied and complementary techniques of canning, freezing and dehydration. Without food additives consumer choice would be severely restricted.

In 1957 the Joint FAO/WHO Expert Committee on Food Additives recognised the advantages to the consumer of the appropriate use of food additives as the maintenance of nutritional quality, the enhancement of keeping quality and reduction of waste, making food attractive, and aiding food processing (FAO/WHO, 1957).

The Committee also stressed the need for ensuring the safety of food additives and regulating their use. Activity in these areas has increased enormously in the last decade. Large resources of money and skilled scientific manpower are currently being devoted to the safety evaluation of food additives and elaborate machinery exists, at the national and international levels, to control their application in practice. In 1962 the British Industrial Biological Research Association (BIBRA) was set up by the British food and allied industries, with government support, to screen substances used or proposed for use in food and carry out basic studies in the methodology of toxicological evaluation. That BIBRA has trebled its size in ten years is an indication of the importance attached to food additives by both government and industry.

Cyclamate was lost to the industry in circumstances of somewhat exaggerated public alarm, and several other useful compounds have been threatened. The development of new food additives is a costly business and the rewards are uncertain. To normal research and development costs must be added the cost of safety evaluation, which could be anything from £50 000 to £250 000 or more without any guarantee as to the outcome.

If in addition to commercial uncertainties it is felt that additives may be banned on what seems to be incomplete or inadequate evidence, or for reasons that owe more to emotion or expediency or economic considera- tions than to science, industry must hesitate to devote resources to the search for new additives to meet technological needs. It would not be in the interest of the food manufacturer or the consumer if the supply of useful new compounds were to dry up.

Novel proteins

The rapid development in recent years of new protein sources to replace animal protein foods has implications that are as important for nutritionists as they are for the food industry.

Meat simulants made from conventional vegetable sources are now commercially available. Production in the United States, which is mainly from soya beans, has been greatly stimulated by the acceptance of approved products for use in school meals (Ministry of Agriculture, Fisheries and Food, 1972b). In the United Kingdom, a protein isolate from the field bean, *Vicia faba* L., is being produced on a significant scale (Lord Rank Research Centre, 1971). The novelty of these products, which are generally referred to as textured vegetable proteins, lies not in their origin but in the processes by which they are given a meat-like texture and appearance. This is usually accomplished either by extruding a dough through dies under controlled conditions to form chunks or other discrete forms, or by spinning a protein isolate into fibres that can be assembled into chewable pieces.

An entirely different approach to the production of novel proteins is by growing microorganisms on industrial by-products or waste materials as substrates. Two processes for the production of single cell (microbial) proteins have reached or are nearing commercial application in the United Kingdom. In the British Petroleum process (Shacklady, 1972; Gounelle de Pontanel, 1972) special strains of yeast are grown on either pure n-alkanes or a standard refinery gas oil in the presence of nutrients and air as a source of oxygen. Protein from this process is intended at the present stage for use in animal feeds only. In the Ranks Hovis McDougall process (Spicer, 1971) protein is produced by microfungi; currently this is being done by growing *Fusarium* spp. on a substrate of field bean starch.

The nutritional value and the safety in use of novel proteins have been extensively investigated and much work is still in progress. The Ministry of Agriculture, Fisheries and Food has established a Novel Protein Intelligence Unit to monitor developments in this area. The use in food of unconventional sources of protein is currently under review by the Food Standards Committee.

It has been objected (Anonymous, 1972a) that novel proteins are unnecessary in the United Kingdom where there is no lack of dietary protein and that developing countries cannot afford them. The scale on which industrial resources would have to be diverted before novel proteins could make a significant contribution to world protein supplies would be formidable indeed. In the longer perspective, however, it may be unwise to underrate the importance of new sources of protein not dependent on the conversion of plant to animal protein. World population projections carry their own warning.

Nutritional labelling

Partly perhaps as a consequence of the White House Conference on Food, Nutrition and Health (1969), there has been an increasing trend in the United States, with certain types of food products, towards quite detailed declaration on the label of the quantities of nutrients that they contain. The Federal Food and Drug Administration (1973a) has published proposals to regulate the form in which such declarations are made and generally to encourage this practice. The basic principles of these proposals are that when nutrients are declared the amounts of energy, protein, carbohydrate, fat, vitamins and minerals shall be expressed by reference to servings of the food and to officially specified recommended daily allowances for protein, vitamins and minerals. Nutritional labelling in accordance with these principles is to be voluntary except where nutrients are added to the food or nutritional claims are made, but the official view is that competitive pressures will eventually cause most United States food manufacturers to fall in line.

In the United Kingdom, under the terms of the Labelling of Food Regulations 1970, the amounts of energy, vitamins and minerals present in a food need only be stated if claims based on these are made. Where slimming claims are made the energy content of a specified amount of the food must be stated. The carbohydrate and energy contents of diabetic foods must also be declared. When tonic, restorative or medicinal properties are claimed the amount of the 'substance' (which could be a nutrient) present on which the claim is based must be stated. There is nothing in principle to stop manufacturers from giving information about the nutrient composition of their products, but it should be noted that the statutory declarations just described cannot under the present Regulations be made by reference to servings (except possibly in relation to slimming claims) or to recommended daily requirements. It seems likely that nutritional labelling for appropriate categories of foods on a voluntary basis will develop in this country. There is some evidence from United States experience (Food and Drug Administration, 1972) that nutritional labelling can increase sales, but whether this would be true in the British market is unknown. At present only a small minority of consumers appear to want to read labels in detail but perhaps with rising educational standards, and a growing awareness of the significance of nutrition for health, habits can be expected to change in the course of time.

Health foods

A health food has been defined as 'any food that retains all its nutritionally desirable constituents and has not had added any substance that is harmful'

(Sinclair, 1972) but this definition hardly does justice to the wide range of criteria by which producers of health foods seek to distinguish their products. Emphasis is frequently placed on production without the use of artificial fertilisers or agricultural chemicals such as pesticides and herbicides and on freedom from food additives. Foods produced under natural ('free range') conditions are another popular class of health foods, as well as 'unrefined' foods such as whole grain cereal products and raw sugar.

Sales of health foods were estimated in 1970 at £18 m, minute in relation to the total market but growing at a rate of 20% per year (Economist Intelligence Unit, 1971). It is entirely proper that those who dislike intensive methods of animal husbandry should be able to buy foods produced by more traditional methods. If consumers prefer to eat unprocessed foods, or believe that compost-grown foods taste better than those produced by conventional methods, there is no reason why they should not spend their money in this way. It is unfortunate, however, that health food publicity is frequently coloured by suggestions that conventional (?unhealthy) foods are less safe and less nutritious. I am unaware of any serious evidence to support either proposition. The long list of toxicants that may occur naturally in food (Food Protection Committee, Food and Nutrition Board, 1967) is a reminder that 'natural' foods are not themselves safe *per se*. It is paradoxical that the exaggerated and misleading claims made for some health foods (McLachlan, 1972) appear to be immune from the statutory and voluntary controls that apply to product claims based on research. It is to be hoped that the more specific controls of tonic, restorative and medicinal claims in the Labelling of Food Regulations 1970 that came into force on January 1 1973 will introduce some discipline in this area.

Dietary fibre

During the last half century the total amount of fibre in the British diet appears to have changed very little but the proportion derived from cereals has fallen (Robertson, 1972).

Medical opinion as to the importance of fibre (or roughage) in the diet has varied over the years. Habitual ingestion of low roughage diets was commonly blamed for constipation in the first half of the century, but by 1956 it was stated in a standard textbook (Mottram and Graham, 1956) that 'the value of ... "roughage" in the diet has been, and still is, overrated'. More recently, interest has revived in a possible association between low fibre diets and a variety of diseases prevalent in modern western society.

Burkitt (1972, 1973) has reviewed a body of mainly epidemiological evidence to suggest that a lack of dietary fibre, and particularly cereal fibre, may be a common causal factor in diverticulosis coli, appendicitis, neoplasms of the large intestine, ulcerative colitis, cholesterol gallstones, coronary heart disease, varicose veins, haemorrhoids, deep vein thrombosis, hiatus hernia, diabetes, obesity and dental caries. A causal relationship between low fibre diets and any of these diseases has yet to be established and it is of course not suggested that a lack of fibre is solely responsible. Nevertheless, if it were eventually to be demonstrated that a deficiency in dietary fibre played even a minor role in their aetiology this could have implications for important sectors of the food processing industry, especially those concerned with cereal products.

Obesity

Although the aetiology of obesity is not fully understood, medical opinion is unanimous in associating excess body fat with ill-health and reduced life expectancy (Office of Health Economics, 1969). Public awareness of these problems, coupled with aesthetic considerations, has generated a unique degree of interest in this widespread nutritional disorder and especially with dietary measures to control it. This situation presents problems for those whose business it is to sell food.

Manipulation of the proportions of carbohydrate, fat and protein in the diet appears to have little effect long term on bodyweight (Pilkington, 1960; Kinsell *et al.*, 1964) but the possibility that dietary sucrose may be more fattening than are other carbohydrates (Allen and Leahy, 1966; Brook and Noel, 1969; Macdonald and Taylor, 1972) has yet to be fully investigated in man. Most reducing diets, whether professionally prescribed or self-imposed, are based on restriction of carbohydrate intake. A wide range of unsweetened or saccharin sweetened low energy foods, as well as starch-reduced foods, is marketed. The ban on cyclamates in 1969 has made it more difficult to formulate palatable sugarless foods, and it is to be hoped that alternative energy-free sweeteners will be developed before long. Other foods to aid dieters depend on presentation in convenient units of specified energy content. The claims that can be made for foods for use in slimming are strictly controlled by the Labelling of Food Regulations 1970 as well as by restrictions on advertising under the terms of the Television Act 1964 and the Sound Broadcasting Act 1972 and through the voluntary controls operated under the aegis of the Advertising Standards Authority.

Dental caries

The predominant environmental factors that determine the onset of this disease, which is virtually endemic throughout the western world, are dietary and microbiological. The carious lesion is initiated by acid generated by bacterial degradation of dietary carbohydrate (Miller, 1890; Graf and Mühlemann, 1966). The level of caries can be reduced by restricting the amount and frequency of ingestion of carbohydrate, especially in the form of sticky, sweet foods that tend to be retained in the mouth. In the absence of any real prospect of reforming public dietary habits in this regard, possible alternative measures to control dental caries have been extensively investigated. The incidence of caries among children (WHO, 1972) and adults (Murray, 1971) can be greatly reduced by adjusting the fluoride ion level of the public water supply to 1 ppm, but efforts to introduce this relatively simple measure of public health nutrition have encountered strong resistance and currently only 5% of the UK population are being supplied with fluoridated water. Attempts to provide fluoride by addition to various foods (Hodge and Smith, 1970) have met with only limited success. Although any fermentable carbohydrate can apparently contribute to the carious process in man, there is much epidemiological, clinical and biochemical evidence to suggest that sucrose is especially cariogenic (Gustafsson et al., 1954; Winter, 1968; Johnson, 1969; Hartles, 1971). There would appear to be scope for reformulation of food with less cario-genic sugars such as glucose syrups (Birch et al., 1970) or with non-caloric sweeteners (Brook, 1970, 1971). A low acidity glucose syrup ascorbic acid product for children introduced in 1966 failed commercially, but this was partly in my view for want of adequate professional support. As with low energy foods the loss of cyclamates has hampered development in this area.

Coronary heart disease

There is now abundant evidence that dietary fat is a factor in the aetiology of this disease, which is a major cause of death in most western countries. Epidemiological, experimental and clinical studies have clearly demon-strated that a positive correlation exists between the level of plasma cholesterol and the incidence of coronary heart disease (Keys, 1970). It has been shown many times that blood cholesterol levels can be reduced by substituting polyunsaturated fat for saturated fat in the diet (see for example National Diet—Heart Study Research Group, 1968). Last autumn the National Academy of Science—National Research Council and the American Medical Association (1972) in a joint statement declared that 'the evidence now available is sufficient to discourage further temporizing . . .'. They recommended that people with elevated levels of plasma lipids, especially cholesterol, should replace part of the saturated fat in their diets with polyunsaturated vegetable oils. They further recom-mended that foods useful for this purpose should be readily available and appropriately labelled. Any regulatory barriers to the marketing of such foods should be removed. Food manufacturers have not been slow to respond to accumulating evidence of the dietary value of polyunsaturated fats in relation to this multifactorial disease. Some had the courage to move well before medical advice could be firm. It might be said that the industry has to a degree anticipated therapeutic need. Thus margarines with excellent organoleptic properties are available which contain 50%

or more of *cis cis* linoleic acid (van Stuyvenberg, 1969). An interesting recent development is that polyunsaturated margarine is now available in New Zealand on prescription (Anonymous, 1972b). Following a recommendation by the National Heart Foundation of New Zealand (1971) that polyunsaturated margarines and spreads should be freely available, especially to those with elevated blood cholesterol levels, measures have been taken to allow people with an appropriate medical certificate to buy up to NZ $20 worth of margarine a year. This is an important modification of the severe restrictions on the importation into New Zealand of products that might threaten the dairy industry. Growing interest in the dietary use of polyunsaturated fats is reflected in proposals by the Food and Drug Administration (1973b) that will allow more information to be given about cholesterol and fat content on food labels.

The role of dietary carbohydrate, and especially of dietary sucrose, in the aetiology of coronary heart disease is less clear. Yudkin and Roddy (1964) and Yudkin and Morland (1967) reported higher sucrose intakes among patients who had survived a myocardial infarction than among controls but this apparent association has not been substantiated by other investigators (Medical Research Council, 1970). Increased sucrose consumption tends to raise serum triglyceride levels but the response varies with the sex of the consumer, the type of dietary fat eaten and other factors (Macdonald, 1970, 1972). The significance of carbohydrate-induced hyperlipidaemia in relation to coronary heart disease is, moreover, still uncertain. Thus there is at present insufficient information available to enable the value of restricting dietary sucrose in reducing the risk of coronary heart disease to be fully assessed.

Associations have been suggested between softness of the water supply and cardiovascular mortality (Crawford, 1972) and between the level of dietary sodium chloride intake and the onset of hypertension (Dahl, 1972). Here also the relevance, if any, of these findings for the food manufacturer remains to be elucidated.

CONCLUSIONS

In many different areas the operations and indeed the structure of the food industry have been profoundly influenced, directly or indirectly, by nutritional science. The growing recognition that food science and technology and nutrition are closely allied disciplines will help to ensure that nutrition continues to play an appropriate role within the industry. There already exists a wide range of foods produced to meet nutritional needs or for use in the management of nutritional disorders. Advances in nutrition are sure to show the need for new formulations and for changes in existing products. Problems arising from the technology and safety evaluation of food additives will require continuing cooperation between government and industry for their solution. Growing world populations must inevitably stimulate demands for new food sources and the better utilisation of existing resources. More regulatory activity in relation to nutrition can be expected, but this should cause no difficulties for a science-based industry so long as innovation is not unnecessarily restricted. Public interest in nutrition and increasing government involvement in nutritional standards will present new challenges to the industry that I am confident will be met.

REFERENCES

Allen, R. J. L. and Leahy, J. S. (1966). *Br. J. Nutr.*, **20**, 339.
Allen, R. J. L., Barker, J. and Mapson, L. W. (1944). *Proc. Nutr. Soc.*, **1**, 129.
Anonymous (1972*a*). *Lancet*, **2**, 1012.
Anonymous (1972*b*). *Fd. Proc.*, No. 12, 5.
Birch, G. G., Green, L. F. & Coulson, C. B. (editors) (1970). *Glucose Syrups and Related Carbohydrates*, Applied Science, London.
Brook, M. (1970). *Dent. Hlth*, July/September, 46.
Brook, M. (1971). In *Sugar*, p. 32, edited by J. Yudkin, J. Edelman and L.
Brook, M. and Noel, P. (1969). *Nature, Lond.*, **222**, 562.
    Hough, Butterworth, London.
Burkitt, D. P. (1972). *Br. Nutr. Fdn Bull.*, No. 7, 29.
Burkitt, D. P. (1973). *Br. med. J.*, **1**, 274.
Central Statistical Office (1972). *National Income and Expenditure* 1972, HMSO, London.
Crawford, M. D. (1972). *Proc. Nutr. Soc.*, **31**, 347.
Dahl, L. K. (1972). *Am. J. clin. Nutr.*, **25**, 231.
Davidson, S., Passmore, R. and Brock, J. F. (1972). *Human Nutrition and Dietetics*, 5th ed. Churchill Livingstone, Edinburgh and London.
Economist Intelligence Unit (1971). *Retail Business*, No. 163, 26.
FAO/WHO (1957). *FAO Nutr. Mtg Rep. Ser.*, No. 15.
FAO/WHO (1971). *FAO Nutr. Mtg Rep. Ser.*, No. 49.
Food and Drug Administration (1972). *Fed. Reg.*, **37**, 6493.
Food and Drug Administration (1973*a*). *Fed. Reg.*, **38**, 2125.
Food and Drug Administration (1973*b*). *Fed. Reg.*, **38**, 2132.
Food Manufacturers' Federation (1972). Unpublished data.
Food Protection Committee, Food and Nutrition Board (1967). *Toxicants Occurring Naturally in Foods*, National Academy of Sciences—National Research Council, Washington, D.C.
Gounelle de Pontanel, H. (editor) (1972). *Proteins from Hydrocarbons*, Comité Scientifique, Symposium d'Aix-en-Provence, Centre de Recherches Foch, Paris.
Graf, H. and Mühlemann, H. R. (1966). *Helv. odont. Acta*, **10**, 94.
Gustafsson, B. E., Quensel, C.-E., Lanke, L. S., Lundqvist, C., Grahnén, H., Bonow, B. E. and Krasse, B. (1954). *Acta odont. Scand.*, **11**, 232.

Harris, R. S. and von Loesecke, H. (editors) (1960). *Nutritional Evaluation of Food Processing*, The Avi Publishing Co. Inc., Westport, Conn.

Hartles, R. L. (1971). In *Sugar*, p. 221, edited by J. Yudkin, J. Edelman and L. Hough, Butterworth, London.

Hodge, H. C. and Smith, F. A. (1970). In *Dietary Chemicals* vs. *Dental Caries*, p. 93, Advances in Chemistry Series, edited by R. F. Gould, American Chemical Society, Washington, D.C.

Hollingsworth, D. F. and Martin, P. E. (1972). *Wld Rev. Nutr. Diet.*, **15**, 1.

Johnson, N. W. (1969). *Practitioner*, **203**, 49.

Keys, A. (editor) (1970). *Circulation*, 41, Supplement No. 1.

Kinsell, L. W., Gunning, B., Michaels, G. D., Richardson, J., Cox, J. E. and Leman, C. (1964). *Metabolism*, **13**, 193.

Lord Rank Research Centre (1971). *Cerebos NVP—A New Vegetable Protein Isolate for the Food Industry*, Lord Rank Research Centre, High Wycombe.

Macdonald, I. (1970). *Biblthca 'Nutr. Dieta'*, No. 15, 129.

Macdonald, I. (1972). *Clin. Sci.*, **43**, 265.

Macdonald, I. and Taylor, J. (1972). *Proc. Nutr. Soc.*, **31**, 36A.

McLachlan, T. (1972). *Roy. Soc. Hlth J.*, **92**, 57.

Medical Research Council (1970). *Lancet*, **2**, 1265.

Miller, W. D. (1890). *The Micro-Organisms of the Human Mouth*, The S. S. White Dental Manufacturing Co., Philadelphia.

Ministry of Agriculture, Fisheries and Food (1971). *Household Food Consumption and Expenditure*: 1969, HMSO, London.

Ministry of Agriculture, Fisheries and Food (1972*a*). *Food Facts*, No. 22, 9.

Ministry of Agriculture, Fisheries and Food (1972*b*). *Novel Protein Intelligence Unit Bull*, No. 1.

Mottram, V. H. and Graham, G. (1956). Hutchison's *Food and the Principles of Dietetics*, 11th ed., Edward Arnold (Publishers) Ltd, London.

Murray, J. J. (1971). *Br. dent. J.*, **131**, 391.

National Academy of Science—National Research Council and American Medical Association (1972). *Nutr. Rev.*, **30**, 223.

National Diet—Heart Study Research Group (1968). *Circulation*, 37, Supplement, No. 1.

National Heart Foundation of New Zealand (1971). *Coronary Heart Disease*, National Heart Foundation of New Zealand, Dunedin.

Office of Health Economics (1969). *Obesity and Disease*, Office of Health Economics, London.

Office of Population Censuses and Surveys (1972). *Population Projections No. 2, 1971—2011*, HMSO, London.

Pilkington, T. R. E. (1960). *Lancet*, **1**, 856.

Robertson, J. (1972). *Nature, Lond.*, **238**, 290.

Shacklady, C. A. (1972). *Wld Rev. Nutr. Diet.*, **14**, 154.

Sinclair, H. M. (1972). In *Health and Food*, p. 11, edited by G. G. Birch, L. F. Green and L. G. Plaskett, Applied Science, London.

Spicer, A. (1971). *Trop. Sci.*, **13**, 239.

van Stuyvenberg, J. H. (editor) (1969). *Margarine: An Economic, Social, and Scientific History*, 1869–1969, University Press, Liverpool.

White House Conference on Food, Nutrition and Health (1969). *Final Report*, US Government Printing Office, Washington, D.C.
WHO (1972). *Tech. Rep. Ser.*, No. 494.
Winter, G. B. (1968). *Br. dent. J.*, **124,** 407.
Yudkin, J. and Morland, J. (1967). *Am. J. clin. Nutr.*, **20,** 503.
Yudkin, J. and Roddy, J. (1964). *Lancet*, **2,** 6.

PART 6

CONCLUSIONS AND RECOMMENDATIONS

CHAPTER 27

Nutrition research today

A. S. TRUSWELL

Professor of Nutrition and Dietetics, Queen Elizabeth College, London

In opening the penultimate general discussion of this Conference I feel that I should try to draw together the many different strands of ideas that have been produced at our meetings in the last few days.

I can perhaps best do this under the heading of this morning's meeting by considering what seem to be the active areas of research in nutrition in the developed countries such as Britain.

First there are occasional mild to moderate deficiencies of the well-known vitamins. Deficiency states do occur and I believe the chances are they will always be with us as minority problems in ever-changing circumstances. Many people thought, 10 or 15 years ago, that nutritional deficiencies had been eradicated in this country. But it is clear from many contributions to this Conference that some deficiencies can be found today in children, in immigrants, in the sick and the old. The main task for nutritional research is vigilance—to be always on the lookout for new minority groups that may become at risk as social and environmental circumstances change.

In addition to the well-known nutrients, we have to consider the possibility of deficiencies of some new nutrients such as trace elements. Their importance has been well worked out for crops and animals but we are only beginning to discover how human deficiencies can occur and what effects they can have. Zinc is a good example. There were many papers on it at the 1972 International Nutrition Congress in Mexico. Human deficiency has been established in the Middle East—Professor Darby's team were pioneers in this—and it has even been claimed recently that suburban children in the USA may sometimes be affected.

Then (in contrast to the water-soluble vitamins) we are only beginning to understand the biochemistry of the fat-soluble vitamins. It was a privilege to hear several workers reporting measurements of minute amounts of vitamin D metabolites in human specimens. The intense activity in this field originates very largely in the beautiful work that Dr Kodicek has been directing at the Dunn Nutritional Laboratory here in Cambridge. Among many practical applications that have been published in recent months are the mechanisms for calcium disturbances in people with kidney disease and in epileptics taking anti-convulsant drugs.

At the other end of the fat-soluble vitamin group, vitamin E is still shrouded in mystery. We don't understand how it works at the biochemical level, yet its deficiency causes various severe diseases in animals and I would expect we will hear more about it and the other fat-soluble vitamins in coming years.

These deficiency states are, however, only a small part of our nutritional problems in Britain. Labelling of foods with vitamin contents will be misleading if it supports the belief that all we have to do is eat enough vitamins, A, B, C etc. and we shall be all right. We owe a great deal to the hypothesisers who have cried out that there is much more to nutrition than avoiding deficiencies. Men like John Yudkin and, at this Conference, Hugh Sinclair and Denis Burkitt have expounded their own broad visions of the subject and given us many ideas to put to experimental test.

The 1930s and early 1940s were the end of the classical vitamin era. After the Second World War nutritional research throughout the world entered an era of preoccupation with protein nutrition. There was intense investigation of the nutritional quality of different dietary proteins and, starting shortly after, of the effects of different dietary fats on plasma cholesterol. More recently we have been in an era of investigating the nutritional effects of quality of carbohydrates, in which Professor Macdonald was a pioneer. These were absorbable carbohydrates. There are still unanswered questions here but the broad picture is I think becoming clear. The new era we are about to enter is that of investigating the effects of quality of unabsorbable carbohydrates. Mr Burkitt and Dr Southgate have given us the present state of knowledge from their different approaches and there is now much experimental work to be done.

The methodology of testing new drugs for toxicity, which became very sophisticated and comprehensive after thalidomide, is now being applied more and more to new food additives. Some of the same critical approach seems to be extending to our well established natural foods. It is likely that all natural foods may contain small amounts of toxin as well as large amounts of nutrient. These natural toxins may sometimes cause trouble either if we eat very large amounts of a single food or under special circumstances. The latest natural food, which has been under suspicion this last year, is the humble potato. Next year it may be the turn of another traditional food that we take for granted today.

There is now considerable circumstantial evidence that ordinary salt—sodium chloride—the oldest food additive—may not be without undesirable effects on the human body. We heard about large amounts of salt in babies' formulae from Dr Taitz and Dr Widdowson. Added salt may not only be too much for the newborn kidneys, it may also predispose to high blood pressure in later life. We can expect and need more research on this.

People in a prosperous society are likely as they grow older to try to choose environmental conditions which increase their probability of postponing the onset of the common degenerate diseases of later life. This is surely part of a life of quality. And the environment includes what they eat. Coronary heart disease, other vascular diseases, diabetes, gallstones, some cancer, osteoporosis, urinary stones, gout, high blood pressure, diverticulosis, even old age and senility itself—there are clues, or in some cases strong evidence, that the development of these diseases is *partly* determined by the dietary pattern over many years. But there are immense methodological problems because all these diseases are almost certainly multifactorial. Diet is only one factor and they develop very slowly with very long subclinical incubation periods.

There is increasing knowledge about and interest in individual variations in handling food components. I am thinking not so much of the rare inborn errors of metabolism for which, as Professor Allen has told us, the food industry has produced many valuable dietetic specialities. There are a number of more common individual metabolic peculiarities which can give trouble in older people. We have discussed deficiency of lactase in the intestine at this Conference. Most non-Caucasian adults and older children can't split milk sugar into its constituent monosaccharides. It is not yet clear how important this is among the nutritional problems of the developing countries. Favism is a potential hazard and a current problem for the introduction of field bean textured proteins. There could be a small number of immigrants coming from round the Mediterranean who would be made ill by eating *Vicia faba*.

Other common individual metabolic variations like the hyperlipidaemias and the obesities (obesity is presumably a syndrome with several biochemical and physiological types) are being actively investigated at present.

As our foods change—the ways they are grown, manufactured and processed, such as intensive animal husbandry or the Chorleywood bread process—and as our choice of foods changes, nutritionists will have to monitor any possible effects. It is a good start that old foods produced by new processes are being analysed chemically in the Laboratory of the Government Chemist as described by Mr Hubbard. But in some cases biological testing in man would be the ideal safeguard. Among the changing food habits is the current fashion of consuming pharmacological doses of vitamin C. As Professor Sinclair has implied, we will need to be on the watch for toxic effects like oxalate stone formation.

Among other miscellaneous areas of current nutrition research being done are:

1. Nutrition and brain biochemistry—not only brain development in babies but possible effects of nutrition on amines in the brain which could have some relation to mental diseases.
2. The interactions of nutrition and drugs. We have heard from Dr Callender how aspirins may predispose to iron loss and from

Professor Sinclair how oral contraceptives appear to increase pyridoxine requirements. There are many other such interactions already known. And the nutritional status may affect the body's ability to detoxify standard doses of drugs.

3. There is much present interest in the effect of maternal diet during pregnancy on the offspring—not only beneficial nutrient conditions but also teratogenic possibilities in what we eat.

Dr Kodicek suggests nutrition and susceptibility to viral infections and the relation of absorption of macromolecules to auto immunity as other fields which offer great scope for nutrition research.

There is growing realisation that our ability to communicate nutritional concepts and advice has not kept pace with scientific and medical knowledge. We need to know much more of how to change food habits (Professor Yudkin was one of the first to point this out). Those who say you can't change food habits are obviously wrong. The Eskimos or the Masai are not born with their traditional eating habits. If you can't change food habits there would be no point in spending money on television commercials about food. I think the marketing side of the food industry understands much better how to change food habits than do nutritionists, do-gooders, doctors, dietitians and dentists. It is encouraging that Weight Watchers are giving much emphasis to the psychological and communication aspect of weight reducing regimes.

It is not only how to influence change that we must try to improve. Our concepts for teaching nutrition at different levels of complexity are mostly out of date. I don't believe that nutritionists can't produce a consensus of opinion on the best way to feed a child. But we do have difficulty in expressing such a complex answer, depending as it does on biochemical concepts and medical provisos.

I expect that the *methodology* of nutrition research is going to be more human: more biochemical than clinical, more in the community than the ward—and there is a crying need for many medium and long term feeding trials. With experimental animals I believe we have to work out more carefully which are the best experimental models for a particular aspect of nutrition and metabolism. I expect the use of appropriate tissue preparation will continue and probably increase.

Where is the money to come from for the many needs for further human research that almost every speaker at this Conference has pointed out? Since the Second World War most of the imaginative and expensive nutritional trials have been done in the USA, in Scandinavia and even in some of the developing countries. There has been very little British medium to large scale human nutrition research since the days of Krebs and McCance and Widdowson's trials in the 1940s.

A special problem with nutrition in most countries is that responsibility usually falls between several Government departments. This country is no exception. Which Government agency is responsible for providing for nutrition research—the Department of Health and Social Security, the Ministry of Agriculture, Fisheries and Food, the National Health Service, the Medical Research Council, the Agricultural Research Council, the Science Research Council, the Social Science Research Council or the University Grants Committee?

It is sobering to reflect that the cost of a three minute television commercial for a food product is about the same amount of money as most university nutrition departments in this country have for their annual research budgets. The capital investment in human nutrition research has been so inadequate that if any food company wanted to do a medium scale human trial on contract at short notice no one would have the plant or the trained manpower to do it.

CHAPTER 28

Reflections at the conclusion of the conference

W. J. DARBY

President, The Nutrition Foundation, Inc, New York

I wish to express my personal thanks and the appreciation of The Nutrition Foundation for the privilege of attending this stimulating and rewarding Conference. In opening the meeting, the Director of The British Nutrition Foundation noted that it is a *first* in three ways. It is also a first in another way—the visible commencement of meaningful cooperation between the three national Nutrition Foundations, The British Nutrition Foundation, The Swedish Nutrition Foundation and The Nutrition Foundation, Inc. Not only has the meeting catalysed interactions and communications nationally, but it will have an international impact.

This Conference on nutritional problems in a changing world has underscored that written by Francis Bacon '. . . the real and legitimate goal of the sciences is the endowment of human life with new inventions and riches'. To meet the needs of the changing world the fullest use of the sciences must be made '. . . not to make imperfect man perfect . . .' but to make imperfect man comfortable, happy and healthy, and to provide him with those necessities, facilities and pleasures that contribute to the quality of life.

Industrialised societies increasingly seek freedom from subsistence agriculture, menial labour, discomfort and disease. There is an ever increasing shift of the responsibility for food production, preparation and use from the individual or family to industry. It is the components and impacts of this phenomenon that occupy us as we utilise science and technology in our changing world to endow life with Bacon's 'new inventions and riches'.

It is the force and uncertainty of the application of scientific technology that underlies much of the anxiety about the nutritive quality and safety of our food supply or the hidden icebergs of undetected disease, and our sometimes emotional efforts to stem the tide of inevitable change.

Uncertainty due to incomplete knowledge will ever plague the critical scientist, but he must distinguish between *incomplete* knowledge and ignorance or absence of knowledge. The government servant with responsibility for formulation of regulations and of governmental policy and the industrial scientist or the industrial executive must make decisions based upon existing information and educated judgments of calculated benefits, costs and risks. Some of the debate of this Conference suggests that not all appreciate this.

There is inherent risk in all facets of living, and benefits to be gained from assuming the risks. The magnitude of each and the accuracy with which they can be assessed range widely.

Similarly, the degree of certainty to which one can approximate an absolute biological concept such as requirement, biological availability, the most desirable growth rate or nutriture varies so widely that often the approximate represents but a 'best judgment for the present'—yet upon such judgments must rest decisions, even if the decision is one to take no action. When this is the case, the decision maker must weigh the consequence of no action versus action based upon the existing judgment of benefits and risks or costs. Is it better to increase the dietary intake of a nutrient to a level judged to meet the highest physiological requirement in the population, even though one knows that the increase will not cure deficiencies of non-dietary origin? Does the possibility of improved nutrition of the pregnant woman, her foetus and the lactating woman and nursing child justify the measure? Such decisions must be made and based upon judgments—judgments that require the counsel of a diverse group of scientists.

It is precisely toward such judgments and decisions that The British Nutrition Foundation can make a major contribution. Indeed, it has made one through this meeting that has brought together scientists from diverse backgrounds and institutions for days of useful dialogue.

During this meeting there have been identified certain areas of scientific and public concern that profitably may serve as a focus of future study by smaller committees of mixed professional composition. Infant feeding and the formulation and use of infant foods (including consideration of how to educate the mother) is one that should be given high priority for continuing joint consideration by a group of paediatricians and nutritional and food scientists from the academic, industrial and governmental communities.

Other areas that strike one as deserving like attention include surveillance of food and nutritional status and interpretation of its findings; the improvement of feeding of the elderly; and the study of food composition— the composition of our changing food. No doubt additional topics can be identified.

But to return momentarily to surveillance, such a committee might well consider the objectives, needs and ultimate use of differing types of data, especially for planning desirable nutritional measures to be taken by the food industry. The design of future products with the increasing trends towards convenience foods and food analogues should follow sound nutritional guidelines that could be developed by such a committee.

The responsibility for surveillance is a multiple one and it requires a coordinated system of information gathering and analysis—a system that includes national and local governmental resources, members of the academic community, the medical profession and industry. Interested participation of physicians in nutritional surveillance of persons with diseases or conditions that produce nutritional risks could greatly promote understanding of nutrition by the medical profession, as well as add to our knowledge of nutritional needs. The industry has much to contribute to this subject in terms of marketing information and their data on changing use patterns of types of products. Similarly, they have much to contribute to revised compilations of food composition. And they are the direct medium for effecting certain needed changes of nutrient intake through any desirable enrichment or fortification, through formulation of products and through alterations in types of ingredients where such is determined to be in the best interest of the public.

A subject not discussed in relation to surveillance, but which is of utmost importance in our changing world is the necessity for establishing and monitoring acceptable levels of beneficial additives in the diet and allowable levels of contaminants. The surveillance system should be designed to produce data applicable to these factors in the food supply.

Contacts between scientists from the triad of academia, industry and government and the direct communication that results from jointly considering important nutritional matters goes far to destroy the barriers that traditionally exist. In our changing world it is essential that these barriers be lowered. Mutual understanding and respect are necessary in a technologically developed society.

Often I have thought that the leading food industry corporations could usefully codify that industry's concepts of corporate responsibility and of corporate citizenship in a code that would be concerned with nutritional values, wholesomeness and safety of food products, advertising claims and competitive comparisons, and the promotion of sound nutritional concepts in corporate advertising. I know many companies that have corporate policy statements of this sort for internal guidance, but I am suggesting a public code for the whole of the industry—indeed last year at Vienna a similar suggestion was put forth by Mr Howard Harder of CPC International who challenged the industry to develop such an international code of ethics. This might well be a subject worthy of exploration by our respective Nutrition Foundations. Voluntary adherence to an appropriately considered publicly stated code would minimise the imposition of new restrictions and would give assurance to the consumer that might prevent his unjustified attacks on the integrity of the food supply—attacks that have become so common in at least my country. Increased consumer confidence could lead to more sound and thoughtful attitudes or demands relating to other developments, such as labelling.

Reflection on the broad implications of this meeting leads me to suggest that a similar future one might address some of the problems of communication between scientists and the non-scientific community, especially relative to decision making, policy, and the quality of life. Recently I expressed the view that: 'Scientists alone cannot make decisions and enforce policy. Value judgments seldom if ever are founded upon science and strict logic. They cannot be made solely upon nutritional or indeed even toxicologic considerations. These considerations should enter into formulation of value judgments, but often do not. Value judgments made by individuals or society are composites of attitudes determined by history, by cultural experiences, by religious and ethical influences, by economic forces, and by needs. They vary with social grouping and with time. They determine the personal satisfaction of the individual and condition his "way of life". It is only recently that scientific considerations have consciously entered into the making of such judgments.

'Accordingly, it is only recently that scientific considerations have entered into formulation of policy and of political decisions. Simultaneously, the nature of forces that influence decisions has dramatically changed because of the immediacy of modern communication media—print, radio and television.

'The complexities of meshing the professional responsibilities of chemists, physicians, food scientists, agriculturalists, industry economists, consumer spokesmen, politicians and statesmen, as well as others, are great. They require tolerance, trust and understanding from all quarters, without which the quality of life open to man through the application of science will not be attained.'

Since policy decisions and legislating actions are politically influenced, indeed laws are enacted by political leaders, it is constructive to consider with Mees (1946) the attitudes and responsibilities of the scientist and the political leader:

'The cleavage in intellectual outlook and mental habits between the political leader and the scientist, the engineer, or, for that matter, the industrialist is a very real and fundamental one and is by no means to be dismissed summarily. It is common for scientists and industrialists to discuss the methods of the politician as if he were either merely stupid or deliberately wicked, while the views of the political expert on the "intellectuals" are often scornful in the extreme.

'As long as men's actions are controlled by their emotions, an objective thinker who discusses every proposition without emotion can have no part in modern political life, since a politician must understand the effect of emotional thought and must be prepared to utilise emotional appeal if he is to obtain popular support. A successful political leader must tend, therefore, either to believe his own emotional appeal or to become a cynic and to some extent a hypocrite if he exerts that appeal without belief. . . .

The appeal to emotion is unavoidable if popular sanction is to be obtained, and yet their critics and often they themselves in retrospect feel that appeal to be false and unwarranted. For this reason alone the political arena would seem to be unsuitable for the scientific man, and those who believe most fully in the value of the scientific spirit should be prepared to understand and sympathise with leaders who must obtain general popular approval for their actions.'

Again, I assert that mutual understanding and respect by all groups is essential if we are to attain Bacon's '. . . real and legitimate goal of the sciences . . . the endowment of human life with new inventions and riches'. I am certain that I speak for all here when I express again our gratitude to The British Nutrition Foundation for its leadership in promoting through this Conference such mutual understanding.

REFERENCE

Mees, C. E. K. (1946). *The Path of Science*, John Wiley and Sons, Inc., New York.

CHAPTER 29

Report by the editors about the conference recommendations

During the Conference several members made suggestions for action by The British Nutrition Foundation and after considerable discussion those present at the final session agreed that written recommendations should be sent in the names of their authors to all members of the Conference for their consideration and, if possible, approval. Those present agreed further that, depending on the views expressed eventually by absent members of the Conference, the recommendations, or modified versions of them, should be made to the Council of the Foundation.

Six recommendations were proposed and are summarised below:

ARTIFICIAL FEEDING OF INFANTS

Six members of the Conference stated that they think breast feeding is optimal for infants aged 0–3 months and expressed concern at the excessive osmolal load relative to water intake from most infant milks mainly because of excessive intakes of protein and sodium. They stated that excessive osmolal load may lead to hypertonic dehydration; thirst and overfeeding; and a theoretical risk of later hypertension. They also expressed the opinion that the addition of cereals and other prepared foods to the diets of infants aged 0–3 months has no proven advantage but contributes to obesity and potential osmolal overload.

They made recommendations that steps should be taken to avoid these risks. They pointed out that one cause of overfeeding is the tendency of mothers to overfill the scoops supplied for the measurement of dried milk for infant feeds.

Proposers

G. C. Arneil   Titular Professor of Child Health, Royal Hospital for Sick Children, Yorkhill, Glasgow G3 8SJ.

Mavis Gunther   77, Ember Lane, Esher, Surrey KT10 8EG.

June K. Lloyd   Institute of Child Health, 30, Guilford Street, London WC1N 1EH

J. C. L. Shaw   Department of Paediatrics, University College Hospital Medical School, Huntley Street, London WC1E 6DH.

C. E. Stroud   Professor of Child Health, King's College Hospital Medical School, Denmark Hill, London SE5 8RX.

L. S. Taitz   The Children's Hospital, Western Bank, Sheffield S10 2TH.

CHILD DEVELOPMENT

One member suggested the establishment of a permanent nutritional survey of child development continuing into adulthood to seek to determine the relationship between early nutrition and health.

Proposer
T. G. Taylor   Professor of Applied Nutrition, Department of Physiology and Biochemistry, The University of Southampton, Southampton SO9 5NH.

ADULT BODYWEIGHT

One member recommended that more research should be done on nutritional factors which affect energy balance, adult bodyweight and the fat content of the body.

Proposer
G. R. Hervey   Professor of Physiology, The University, Leeds LS2 9JT.

AGEING

Two members proposed that, with a view to assessing the influence of nutrition on ageing, attention should be given to the means of assessing nutritional status of the individual and to the development of a battery of tests for measuring biological age.

Proposers
A. N. Exton-Smith   Physician, Geriatric Department, St Pancras Hospital, University College Hospital, 4, St Pancras Way, London NW1 0PE.

B. E. C. Nordin   Director, Medical Research Council Mineral Metabolism Unit, The General Infirmary, Great George Street, Leeds LS1 3EX.

NUTRITIONAL LABELLING OF FOODS

Six members recommended that nutritional labelling of foods should not be introduced until meaningful nutritional recommendations can be made and accepted. They expressed the view that claims for nutrients should be made only for ingredients that are to be ingested. As an example they suggested that a claim for vitamin C added to the liquor for canning potatoes should not be allowable.

Proposers

J. B. M. Coppock	Director of Research and Scientific Services, Spillers Limited, Old Change House, 4–6, Cannon Street, London EC4M 6XB.
J. Green	General Manager, Research and Development Division, H. J. Heinz Company Limited, Hayes Park, Hayes, Middlesex.
H. R. Hinton	Director, The Campden Food Preservation Research Association, Chipping Campden, Glos. GL55 6LD.
A. W. Holmes	Director, British Food Manufacturing Industries Research Association, Randalls Road, Leatherhead, Surrey.
A. Spicer	Director of Research, RHM Research Limited, The Lord Rank Research Centre, Lincoln Road, High Wycombe, Bucks.
F. Wood	Development Director, CPC (United Kingdom) Ltd., Claygate House, Esher, Surrey KT10 9PN.

EDUCATION OF NUTRITIONISTS

Two members pointed out that the adequate future of the science of nutrition can be preserved only if a sufficient number of experts in nutrition are trained. They stated that a satisfactory career structure for nutritionists should be established. They recommended as a means of realising this the formation within the Foundation of a study group with industrial and scientific membership and including representatives of medical schools.

Proposers

E. Kodicek	Director, Dunn Nutritional Laboratory, Milton Road, Cambridge CB4 1XJ.
A. S. Truswell	Professor of Nutrition and Dietetics, Queen Elizabeth College, Atkins Building, London W8 7AH.

Index

Acidosis, obesity and, 19
Addison's disease, 215
Adenosine triphosphate from
    different sources, 162
Adipocytes,
    lipid release from, 25
    multiplication of, 31
    number following fasting, 25
    obesity, in, 23
    storing insulin, 25
Adipose tissue, fat in, 23
Advertising Standards Authority, 260
Ageing, biological tests for, 296
Albumin, plasma levels, 74
Aldosterone, 215
Algal sources of lipids, 169
Alkaline phosphatase, 55, 56
Alpha amylase, action on starch, 1, 95
Alpha-glycerophosphate oxidase, 26
American Heart Association,
        statement on diet and heart
        disease, 183
Amino Acids,
    mobilisation of, 168
    single cell protein, in, 180
    novel proteins, in, 252
p-Aminobenzoic acid, 97
Amylopectin, 194
Anaemia,
    elderly, in, 224
    incidence of, 55
        Czechoslovakia, in, 67
    iron deficiency, 60, 73, 206
    women, in, 55, 67
Appendicitis, dietary fibre and, 37
Ascorbic acid, See Vitamin C

Atherosclerosis, See also Coronary
        heart disease and
        Cardiovascular disease
    fats in aetiology, 184, 186, 190
    relation to nutrition, 66
Australia, National Heart Foundation
        statement on diet and heart
        disease, 189

Bacteria, protein from, 181, 271
Banana, 202
Beans, protein from, 178, 251
Beef, 244, 254
Beef cattle,
    muscle composition, 243, 244
    nutrients in liver, 245
Bile acids, reabsorption of, 35
Birth size, factors involved, 137
Birthweight,
    low, 56
    poverty and, 72
    very low
        See Very low birthweight
        infants
Blood sugar levels in diabetes, 14
Bodyweight, 296
    dangerous, 15, 16
    gain in artificially fed infants, 129
    loss, insulin sensitivity and, 22
    safe, 15, 188
    tables of, 16
Bone loss, calcium in diet and, 217
Bowel function, dietary fibre and, 36
Brain,
    biochemistry and nutrition, 285